Student-Athlete
Meeting the Challenges of College Life

Carl I. Fertman, PhD, CHES
University of Pittsburgh

JONES AND BARTLETT PUBLISHERS
Sudbury, Massachusetts
BOSTON   TORONTO   LONDON   SINGAPORE

World Headquarters

Jones and Bartlett Publishers
40 Tall Pine Drive
Sudbury, MA 01776
978-443-5000
info@jbpub.com
www.jbpub.com

Jones and Bartlett Publishers Canada
6339 Ormindale Way
Mississauga, Ontario L5V 1J2
Canada

Jones and Bartlett Publishers International
Barb House, Barb Mews
London W6 7PA
United Kingdom

Jones and Bartlett's books and products are available through most bookstores and online booksellers. To contact Jones and Bartlett Publishers directly, call 800-832-0034, fax 978-443-8000, or visit our website www.jbpub.com.

Substantial discounts on bulk quantities of Jones and Bartlett's publications are available to corporations, professional associations, and other qualified organizations. For details and specific discount information, contact the special sales department at Jones and Bartlett via the above contact information or send an email to specialsales@jbpub.com.

This publication is designed to provide accurate and authoritative information in regard to the Subject Matter covered. It is sold with the understanding that the publisher is not engaged in rendering legal, accounting, or other professional service. If legal advice or other expert assistance is required, the service of a competent professional person should be sought.

Production Credits

Acquisitions Editor: Jacqueline Ann Geraci
Production Manager: Julie Champagne Bolduc
Editorial Assistant: Kyle Hoover
Production Editor: Tracey Chapman
Production Assistant: Roya Millard
Marketing Manager: Jessica Faucher
Manufacturing Buyer: Therese Connell

Composition: Auburn Associates, Inc.
Photo Research Manager/Photographer: Kimberly Potvin
Cover Design: Brian Moore
Cover Image: © Jones and Bartlett Publisher. Photographed
  by Kimberly Potvin
Printing and Binding: Malloy, Inc.
Cover Printing: Malloy, Inc.

Library of Congress Cataloging-in-Publication Data

Fertman, Carl I., 1950–
  Student-athlete success: meeting the challenges of college life / Carl Fertman.
    p. cm.
  Includes bibliographical references.
  ISBN-13: 978-0-7637-5044-2 (pbk.)
  1. College athletes—United States 2. College sports—United States. I. Title.
  GV351.F37 2009
  796.04′3—dc22

                                                                                    2008011536

6048
Printed in the United States of America
12 11 10 09 08   10 9 8 7 6 5 4 3 2 1

The book is dedicated to
Gabriel, Naomi, Julian, Andy, Jean, and Peter

Contents

Preface

Student-athletes are extraordinary people. On campus, they are the most easily identifiable group of individuals. They are known by people they have never met and are held to high standards. They are expected to balance their academic, athletic, career, personal, and community responsibilities while showing character, integrity, and leadership skills.

Student-athletes need support and help from parents, coaches, professors, and athletic directors to flourish. However, not all student-athletes are successful. Some run into academic challenges, and the demands of getting a college degree take precedent over athletic commitments. For others, the physical demands of practice and competition and lack of proper sleep can, at times, undermine a student-athlete's best intentions to attend class and to study. Physical injuries can often prevent full classroom and athletic participation. Sometimes, the demands of classes and athletics result in unhealthy choices involving drugs, alcohol, violence, and sex.

Student-Athlete Success: Meeting the Challenges of College Life helps student-athletes succeed in meeting the physical, mental, and emotional demands of classes and athletics using a four-pronged approach: frank discussion, self-assessment, accurate information, and action steps to meet goals. This book is an important guide for undergraduate students who are in programs and courses dedicated to working with student-athletes in the fields of health and physical education, sports management, athletic training, health promotion, and sports medicine. This book is also an essential read for coaches, athletic directors, and administrators, as well as parents and high school and college athletes.

Student-Athlete Success: Meeting the Challenges of College Life is based on leading health theories that encourage accurate assessment of an individual's health behavior and motivation to succeed. This book does not assume that college student-athletes have problematic health behaviors, but rather emphasizes that positive health changes can be made if they do have issues. The book goes on to use the four-pronged approach to encourage positive personal development. The topics discussed are truthful and grounded in the student-athlete's personal experience.

Student-Athlete Success: Meeting the Challenges of College Life has four major parts:

- Chapter one explores the route student-athletes must take to become successful in a collegiate setting, including identifying personal goals and the rules to live by (e.g. from NCAA, coaches, and parents). This chapter also focuses on knowing and protecting a student's schedule so they can achieve peak performance in the classroom and on the field.

- Chapter two discusses pressures encountered on and off the field and identifies eight specific challenges that contribute to a student-athlete's overall stress.

- Chapters three through ten are dedicated to each of the eight challenges experienced by collegiate student-athletes: academics, pain and injury, performance enhancers, nutrition, alcohol use and abuse, other substance use and abuse (e.g. marijuana, tobacco and other drugs), sex and relationships, and gambling and money. This section shows student-athletes how to recognize these challenges and learn how to avoid them, to overcome them, to cope with them, and to seek help when necessary.

- Chapter eleven identifies the resources available on and off campus to student-athletes who may need help and support when addressing challenges.

The book's approach is positive and focused on the development of competent and capable student-athletes who perform well in the classroom and on the playing field. It encourages development of positive assets and protective qualities that lead to resilient, caring individuals in both their academic and athletic pursuits.

Key Features:

Learning Objectives

Learning Objectives at the beginning of each chapter focus on the most important concepts to be covered.

Student-Athletes Say

Each chapter opens with a series of comments by real student-athletes.

Student-Athlete Challenge Self-Assessment

Chapters two through ten offer self-assessment activities. Chapter two includes an "Involvement with Challenges" self-assessment that asks student-athletes to assess their level of involvement, whether it is positive or negative, with the eight challenges addressed in this text. All eight "Challenge Chapters" (chapters three through ten) provide self-assessment activities based on an individual's experience with the particular challenge and show whether that experience is positive or negative.

Opening Vignettes

After the initial self assessments, each chapter contains a vignette, written from the perspective of a real student-athlete.

Self-Reflections

Self-Reflections are scattered throughout the chapters and give the reader time to reflect on their level of knowledge, awareness, participation in, and mastery of specific challenge topics.

Think About It

"Think About It" questions at the end of each section within the chapters help the reader to remember what they have read and to apply this knowledge to real-life.

Plugged Into Sports: Student-Athletes and Technology

This special feature highlights the effect and influence that current technology (internet, cell phones, Facebook, and MySpace) has on student-athletes' lives, schedules, and involvement in sports.

Your Thoughts

"Your Thoughts" entries provide opportunities for the reader to express their thoughts in written form. These thoughts are intended to increase self-awareness, improve critical-thinking skills, and apply chapter topics.

Student-Athlete Success: Meeting the Challenges of College Life should be used as a vehicle to talk about issues that are important to student-athletes. Coaches, professors, friends, and family members can get a better understanding of their student-athlete's feelings and can help them use their energy more effectively in the pursuit of their academic and athletic goals.

The college years are times of achievement and success as well as times of anxiety and soul searching. Use *Student-Athlete Success: Meeting the Challenges of College Life* as a guide to help student-athletes make good health decisions and positive health choices while reaching and exceeding their academic and athletic goals.

Acknowledgments

Student-Athlete Success: Meeting the Challenges of College Life is a team effort. I acknowledge and thank for their support Lou Fabian, Dr. Shirley Haberman, Robert Blanc, Tony Salesi, Steve Pederson, Jeff Long, Donna Sanft, Michael Farabaugh, Dr. John Jackicic, Dr. Elizabeth Nagle, Carl Schinasi, Casey Brady Sirochman, Joe Mull, and Jaime Sidani. Thank you to student-athletes Dale Williams, Charles Small, Penny Semaia, and Eric Limkemann and the University of Pittsburgh Student-Athlete Advisory Committee members. Many thanks to Michelle Barbiaux, Shawna Gornlick, Emily Shimko, and Megan McGrane for their work on the manuscript. I would also like to thank Gabriel Fertman, Naomi Fertman, and Andrew Bartholomew for their work and review of a number of chapters. I thank the Maximizing Adolescent Potentials (MAPS) program staff at the University of Pittsburgh for their support. Thank you to Carolyn Simitz for her editing, preparation of the manuscript, and overall good work. My wife, Barbara Murock, the best biker I know, is thanked for her love and support.

Thank you also to the reviewers of this first edition. Their voices, criticism, and support have truly made this a better text:

- Kathy Kaler, Athletic Academic Counselor, Illinois CHAMPS/Life Skills Coordinator; University of Illinois at Urbana-Champaign

- V. Paul Downey, Ed.D, West Virginia University

- Shed Dawson, Jr., B.A., M.P.A., Savannah State University

- Sharon Kay Stoll, Ph.D., Director, Center for ETHICS*; University of Idaho

- Rob Spear, Ph.D, Director of Athletics, University of Idaho

Finally, I appreciate and acknowledge the hundreds of college student-athletes who shared their stories, time, thoughts, and feelings with me which made this book a reality. Every day college student-athletes labor in the classroom and on the playing field to achieve personal goals while bringing visibility, enthusiasm, energy, and excellence to their campus. Thank you.

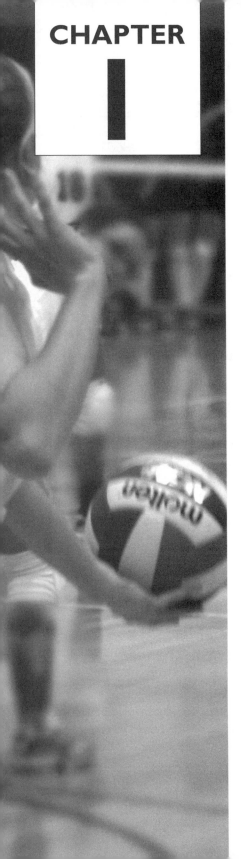

CHAPTER

1

Student-Athletes' Framework for Success

Learning Objectives

After completing this chapter, you will be able to:

- *Reflect on your personal history as both a student and an athlete, and identify the people who have influenced and supported you along the way*

- *Discuss your transition from high school to college and understand new rules and expectations that you have encountered*

- *Identify what you want to get out of being a student-athlete and create your personal agenda*

- *Set short-term and long-term goals for athletics, academics, and life after sports*

Student-Athletes Say:

- I get up at 5:40 A.M. three days a week, and practice twenty hours a week. The time people think we should put into our classes is sometimes unrealistic. I have five classes this semester and they take up a lot of time. I wish everyone realized how much work we put into our sport and our classes.

- After I graduate, no one will care that I could shoot free throws with my eyes closed or that I scored a buzzer beater to win conference playoffs, but hopefully they will care that I'm a determined, dedicated team player who has a good work ethic and values. Playing sports in college taught me a lot, and hopefully employers will recognize this.

- I remember when I first decided that I wanted to be a basketball player. I was watching a game with my dad, and I saw Michael Jordan leap through the air and dunk the ball with one hand. I remember thinking, "I'm going to do that someday."

- I like being part of a team. There is automatically a group of friends by my side who understand everything I am going through.

- Each coach has their own set of rules for their players. For example, my team doesn't have mandatory study halls, while other teams have up to ten hours per week.

- Sometimes I feel like student-athletes have extra pressure and greater expectations placed on them than other students. Everyone knows who we are and people are looking to catch us doing something wrong.

This book is designed to help you, the student-athlete, make healthy decisions in regard to school, sport, and life. It is written to help you meet the challenges that you face and overcome the obstacles that are inherent in the college experience. Before you can learn how to be successful as a student-athlete, it is important that you understand and reflect upon how you came to be a collegiate student-athlete.

Let's start by looking at your student history. By the time you get to college you have a lot of experience being a student. College is different from high school. Besides being older, by the time you reach college you already have knowledge of how school works. Over your previous twelve years of schooling, from elementary school through high school, you have developed attitudes, behaviors, and skills that will carry over into college. The questions in Box 1.1 will help you reflect on these attitudes, behaviors, and skills.

STUDENT REFLECTION
STUDENT REFLECTION

Box 1.1. What Is Your Student History?

1. How was being a student part of your life while you were growing up?

Elementary school	
Middle school	
High school	

2. Growing up, was school fun and interesting? Or was it a chore and boring?

3. Did your parents or guardians help you with your school work?

4. Compared with your friends, how did you do in school?

It may seem that you have been an athlete all of your life. Physical activities and sports were just something you did without even thinking about it. Athletics were a part of life: the same as eating and sleeping. Is it possible that it was all about fun and nourishment? Maybe. Or was it clear from an early age that you thrived on the competition, physical activity, aggression, and emotions that made sports a serious pursuit for you? Box 1.2 provides some questions to help you think about these issues growing up.

Do you see any patterns after working through Boxes 1.1 and 1.2? Perhaps you were always a good student in school without much work. Or maybe you needed to work really hard to get your grades. Maybe you didn't really put much effort into school and realized only in high school that grades and school were important and worth effort. On the sports side, maybe you tried several sports before settling on just one. For many student-athletes, involvement in sports began at an early age and evolved over time, changing as their goals, environment, abilities, and expectations grew.

> *I grew up in a small, rural town. My high school senior class had only a hundred kids, and I was well liked by all of them. I was the captain of the volleyball team and the star middle hitter. I was a big fish in a little pond. College was a huge transition for me. There were thousands of kids at school and I did not know anyone. I arrived on campus early for preseason volleyball and was immediately thrown into a rigorous practice schedule. I felt a little overwhelmed by the level of play; after all, I was no longer the tallest or*

Box 1.2. What Is Your Athletic History?

1. Think back to when you were first exposed to sports. How were physical activity and athletics part of your life while you were growing up?

Elementary school	
Middle school	
High school	
Community/recreational activities	
Family	
Sports you like to watch	

2. Did your parents or guardian coach your team or go to your competition?

3. Did you play multiple sports or focus on just one?

fastest athlete on the team. In a few weeks, my classes began. Now, not only was I busy with volleyball and trying to keep up with my teammates, but I was worried about my classes. I wondered if I would ever feel like I was part of the team. Adding to my stress was my roommate. We did not click. She was very loud and would be up all hours of the night. I could not get any sleep and felt hostility toward her. By fall break, I felt uneasy about everything and was thinking about quitting the team. I felt a great deal of pressure to be a great athlete, fit in with the team, keep up my grades to maintain my scholarship, and please my parents.

In this chapter you will focus on understanding your path to being a college student-athlete and setting your agenda as a college student-athlete. In your college career you are the boss. You set the agenda. It may not always seem that way with so many people telling you what to do and with so many rules to follow. Ultimately, however, you are the person with the responsibility and authority to decide what it is that you want, and how hard you are willing to work to get what you want. It is your choice.

Understanding Your Student-Athlete Journey

You may think that your life as a collegiate student-athlete started when you received a letter of acceptance from your college or university, when you signed a letter of intent, or tried out for and made your athletic team. In reality, your student-athletic career started many years ago. Your long journey, full of hard work and dedication, led to making a college team and possibly even earning an athletic scholarship. Remember the first time you became interested in your sport. Perhaps you saw an elite gymnast on television and watched in awe, or maybe you tried to keep up with your older brother on the soccer field. These events may have seemed insignificant at the time, but they contributed to your development as a student-athlete and helped shape your athletic career. Every athlete has his or her own story. Your story tells how you became interested in sports, why you push yourself to the extreme, and what drives you to compete.

Many factors, experiences, and people shaped your socialization into sport. Your family, community, friends, and coaches played significant roles in your athletic history, shaping your experiences and contributing to challenges and successes in sports. Playing a collegiate sport is an honor that only few receive, and the journey to achieving it is lengthy. Being a successful student-athlete can be very rewarding, but it is not an easy task. This chapter details and discusses the adjustments that occur as you take your involvement in athletics to the next level. It also discusses how you can create your own agenda so that you can continue to have success in school, sport, and life while satisfying your own personal goals and needs.

Adjusting to New Rules and Expectations

Responsibility and Accountability

There are definite advantages to being a student-athlete. However, there are numerous sacrifices and pressures that also come with the territory. In other words, as a student-athlete you have

THINK ABOUT IT

- ❑ What motivates you to be a student-athlete?
- ❑ What do you hope to get out of being a collegiate student-athlete?
- ❑ Many people have helped you become a collegiate student-athlete. Who has influenced your athletic experiences? Who has provided you with encouragement, care, compassion, and understanding along the way?

tremendous opportunities as well as restrictions and responsibility. You have the opportunity to attend college, play the sport you love, and share an experience that few college students have. The tradeoff is that student-athletes must make sacrifices to play their sport. They must abide by rules, give up their free time for practice and games, forgo time with friends, miss out on school breaks, and even miss classes due to their athletic schedules. For most student-athletes, the benefits greatly outweigh the drawbacks; however, sometimes the pressures and demands of playing collegiate sports can become so great that student-athletes begin to question whether playing their sport is worth the tradeoffs.

To gain the privilege of being a student-athlete, you must comply with rules and regulations. The clear consequence of not complying is not playing. The threat of not playing often shapes the way student-athletes behave, act, and comply to the standards set for them. Sometimes it appears that student-athletes are held to higher standards than other college students who do not so openly represent their school, but that is the tradeoff for playing at the collegiate level. Student-athletes are some of the most visible students on campus and in their local community. For this reason, when they put on an athletic uniform, they are representing not only themselves but their team, their sport, and their school. This is a huge responsibility and is not to be taken lightly.

Because you are a part of a larger program and organization, it is important that you uphold the policies, behaviors, and expectations of your institution. Each college and university has its own set of rules and responsibilities that it expects its student-athletes to follow. Rules and expectations range from how you are to handle the media, to how many hours of study hall you attend, to how you are supposed to treat fellow teammates. Typically, schools outline a code of conduct and ethics for their student-athletes to guide them in their decision making and behavior.

A large part of being a student-athlete is dealing with these rules and expectations. They are everywhere. Schools, teams, professors, administrators, parents, guardians, coaches, and the NCAA (National Collegiate Athletic Association) all have their own set of rules and guidelines. At times, it may feel like everyone is trying to restrict what you do or catch you doing something wrong. In reality, the rules are in place to help you better navigate through the rigors of playing a sport, representing your school, being a good student, and having a full and meaningful college experience. A good place to start when discussing rules is to clarify who makes the rules and what they expect from you. Box 1.3 provides an activity to help you think about the rules that are in place in your life. With all the rules that govern collegiate athletics, it is important to be well informed and fully know and understand them. Without knowledge of what is expected and required of you, it is impossible to make good decisions.

Personal Values

As a student-athlete, you have developed your own personal code of values and ethics. How did you do this? The answer is through your relationships with people and how you live your

STUDENT REFLECTION

STUDENT REFLECTION

Box 1.3. Who Rules Your Life?

Think about the people who set rules and have expectations about all that you do in the athletic, academic, personal, and social spheres. Mark (X) the areas where they set rules for you. Give an example of a rule that they impose.

	Athletic	Academic	Social	Personal
Coaches				
Coaches' rules				
School				
School's rules				
NCAA				
NCAA's rules				
Professors				
Professors' rules				
Parents/guardians				
Parents/guardians' rules				
Teammates				
Teammates' rules				
Clergy				
Clergy's rules				
Friends				
Friends' rules				

life—day in and day out. You created your personal values over time. Think about how you interact with people. Do friends and family members value your comments, feedback, and companionship? What personal qualities make you a good person, a person other people want to be with? Likewise, what qualities do you admire and view as worthwhile in your friends, family members, coaches, and teammates? And how do you incorporate those qualities into your daily life?

Your own set of values becomes especially important during the time of transition from high school to college. Chances are, while you were in high school, your parents or guardians set clear rules and expectations for your actions and behaviors. Now that you are in college, you will begin to set your own expectations and boundaries for yourself and your lifestyle. Knowing your personal values and ethics helps you design your own game plan and helps lay out a roadmap for how to make significant choices in your life. Having strong values helps you discover who you are as a person, which in turn results in a personal clarity for

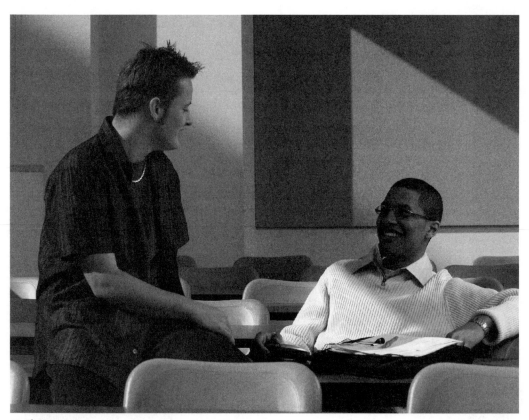

© Photos.com

yourself and other people. Knowing who you are is the first step toward achieving your personal goals and living a self-actualizing existence, while at the same time contributing to your team and school.

Likewise, when thinking about your personal values and ethics, it is important to acknowledge that you have the capability of making an impact on those around you, including teammates, classmates, friends, and prospective college students. In other words, you are in a leadership position. Often, student-athletes are told they are leaders but may not really believe it or understand what it means to be a leader. Leadership takes many forms. Leadership can be displayed through words, actions, beliefs, and everyday way of life. You have the opportunity to be a leader both on and off the playing field. For example, you can lead your team through a tough game by staying calm after a referee makes an unfavorable call. You may also emerge as a leader by giving the team a motivational pep talk during a time out, giving your teammates a better outlook on the game. Because you are so visible on campus, the entire student body is able to observe your dedication to your sport and see the value of hard work. Similarly, every day that you head to class, you set the example that academics and gaining knowledge are things that you value.

Finally, your personal values set a tone for how you conduct yourself. Values such as practicing good sportsmanship and treating others with respect are key components of being a successful student-athlete. Good sportsmanship includes both small gestures and heroic efforts. It starts with something as simple as shaking hands with opponents before a game or accepting a bad call gracefully. Displaying good sportsmanship isn't always easy: It can be tough to congratulate the opposing team after losing a close or important game. Athletes who learn how to be gracious and respectful are class acts and always seem to benefit in the long run.

Rules to Play By

Playing a sport in college means you agree to abide by the NCAA rules and regulations. At the beginning of each school year, you sign an agreement confirming your adherence with the rules as well as understanding of consequences for noncompliance. Every level of organized sport and athletic competition has a governing body. These organizations, including the NCAA, define and regulate all aspects of athletic sports competitions. They regulate eligibility, recruitment, training, officiating, playing rules, and records. If you want to maintain your eligibility as a student-athlete, compliance with all the rules outlined by the NCAA, the governing body of collegiate athletics, is a necessity. The rules established by the NCAA encompass many topics that impact a student-athlete's life. Although the list of rules can be overwhelming, it is important to know them and understand how they apply to you (see Box 1.4).

REFLECTION

STUDENT REFLECTION

Box 1.4. What Are the NCAA Rules?

How well do you know the rules? Read the statements below and identify whether they are true or false.

1. It is not an extra benefit if I use a copy machine in the athletics department for free if I copy less than ten pages.

   False. That is an extra benefit. You may not use any copy machine, fax machine, or telephone for free.

2. I have to be enrolled in twelve credits per semester to be eligible.

   True. In order to be considered "full time" and eligible, you must be enrolled in a minimum of twelve credits each semester.

3. My coach's mandatory study hall hours count toward my weekly total of maximum hours allowed per week.

   False. Study hall hours do not count toward "countable" athletic hours in your week.

4. If I oversleep and miss a scheduled NCAA drug test, it is automatically considered a positive test.

   True. Any missed or skipped NCAA drug test is considered a positive test, pending a retest.

5. When I am in the "off season" I can only participate in ten hours of "countable" athletically related activity.

   False. In the "off season" you are allowed to participate in eight hours of countable athletically related activity.

6. A kid in my class told me he did some gambling and he would give me $500 to close the spread. I said no, because that's illegal. Since I said no, I didn't tell anyone it happened, so this is not a violation.

   False. Although you are not at fault, the NCAA still mandates that you report the person who solicited you to shave points.

7. It is okay to "dip" or use chew tobacco during practice, just not during games since people are watching the games.

   False. Tobacco is not to be used at any time during athletic participation.

8. If you test positive on an NCAA drug test, on the first offense, you get suspended from sport for six months.

   False. A positive NCAA drug test first offense is a twelve-month suspension.

9. My scholarship check is a lot less in the summer but I still stay at school to work out with my teammates. A family that comes to my games said I could live at their house this summer for free, which sounds okay to me.

   False. This is a violation that is considered an extra benefit.

10. You must pass a total of six credits to be eligible for the next semester.

    True. Six credits must be completed for credit in order to remain eligible for competition in the next academic term.

THINK ABOUT IT ✔

❑　What advice would you give to a freshman who is dealing with new rules for the first time as a new college student-athlete?

❑　Since you started college, what rules have changed in your family? On your team? What rules would you change if you were in charge?

❑　Make a list of tradeoffs or sacrifices that you have made to be a student-athlete. Make a separate list of the benefits or perks of being a student-athlete.

❑　Have you ever displayed an act of poor sportsmanship? How did you feel afterward? How would you confront a teammate or opponent who displays poor personal conduct?

You are encouraged to obtain copies and clarification of the NCAA rules and regulations by talking with a member of the coaching staff or a member of the administrative staff. Remember that rules and guidelines are not made to keep you from having fun or enjoying your college experience, but they are put into place to help maintain the integrity and fairness of collegiate athletics, encourage student-athletes to act responsibly, and make sure that all athletes and athletic departments abide by the same principles.

Creating Your Own Agenda

There are academic and athletic responsibilities that come with being a student-athlete such as attending classes, taking credits, and maintaining your grades. In addition, you are required to attend practices, follow the guidelines of good sportsmanship, and keep yourself in elite physical shape. Figuring out how to meet all of these rules and expectations while still fulfilling your own personal goals and ambitions is a challenge that student-athletes face. By understanding the rules in light of your own personal goals, you can be in control of the events in your life despite the pressures you face from classes, coaches, family, and friends.

You are well aware that even during the beginning of your college student-athletic career there are pressures, expectations, and hard work that accompany being a student-athlete. You have to try to live up to expectations of coaches and parents, attend class, follow directions, cope with losing, and work within a team. These are some pretty big expectations to place on a person. With so many pressures and so much hard work, why do people continue to participate in sports in college? Why bother being a student-athlete? Why not just be a student and maybe play intramural sports? Would it make your life easier and a lot less complicated? There are many reasons to be a student-athlete. While student-athletes put a lot of time, energy, and heart into sports, they can also get a lot out of participating. For example, sports shape your lifestyle, friendships, relationships, work ethic, and school participation. Sports may also teach you useful life skills such as teamwork, education, and time management. Sports may also afford you the opportunity to learn from amazing players and coaches, travel, and possibly even further your education in college.

Many student-athletes never take the time to think about why they play sports or what they hope to get out of their participation. This is surprising because no one in their right mind would ever accept a job without finding out what it pays or how they will be compensated, yet student-athletes play every day without defining what is in it for them. Obviously, you cannot be paid to participate in collegiate sports, but there are other things that you could get out of the unique experience. Maybe you play for a scholarship to get an education, maybe you play because you want to make it to the pros and sign a big contract, or maybe you play because of the love you feel for the game or the rush you feel every time you step in the court or on the field. It is important that you understand why you are a student-athlete and going the extra step of playing sports in college—not just being a student but choosing to be a student-athlete.

Part of choosing to be a student-athlete is to set goals for what you wish to accomplish in school and sports. You want to be the star of your collegiate student-athlete career. And to do this you need to create an agenda for what you want to gain and experience as a collegiate student-athlete. Having an agenda means you need to set goals for your college years and beyond.

College Goals

What is a goal? It is a mark, an accomplishment you set your sights on to achieve. Attending all your classes; completing assignments on time; beating your personal best performance in your next practice, competition, or event; increasing your upper-body strength and endurance; creating more scoring opportunities in a game; staying composed when opposing players and fans try to rattle you; getting along better with your roommates; and spending more time with your family over school breaks are examples of common student-athlete goals. Goals give you a focus.

Goals are constantly being reassessed and changed. They are not static; they evolve as circumstances and situations change. As a student-athlete you must constantly check your progress toward reaching your goals and reevaluate your goals in light of your performance, interests, and expectations.

Setting goals can be a great motivator. Make a commitment to yourself that you will take responsibility for your actions and decisions and work to attain your goals. Understand that there will be roadblocks along the way, and do not get discouraged when you encounter obsta-

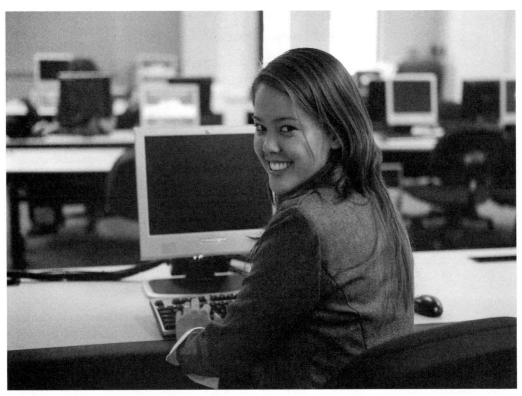

© Stephen Coburn/ShutterStock, Inc.

cles and distractions. Do not let setbacks stop you; set your goals, acknowledge your roadblocks, stick to your plan, and commit yourself to achieving those goals.

You can set goals for yourself in any part of your life. At the beginning of each semester set one or two goals for your sport, classes, social life, and family life. Focus on the current school semester. Take some time to think about what is important to you by completing the exercise in Box 1.5. What do you want to accomplish this semester? It is your choice.

Your team and coaches will also have their own goals for the semester. In establishing your personal goals you will need to consider how your goals match the team's and coaches' goals. Team goals can be met only if all members of the team share the desire to reach that goal. For example, it is useless for a basketball team to have the team goal of making it to the playoffs if the starting forward has his or her personal agenda of learning how to shoot three pointers when the team needs him or her to focus on rebounding. Sharing your goals is an important

REFLECTION

STUDENT REFLECTION

Box 1.5. Set Your College Goals—Current Semester

At the beginning of each semester set one or two goals that you want to accomplish in each area.

Athletic	
Academic	
Social life	
Family life	

part of having them. It is risky to state your goals publicly, but at the same time you can gain support and maybe shape the team goals so your goals match well with your team's and coaches' goals.

Goals Beyond College

It is difficult to set goals and work toward them. In the previous section you set goals for the current school term, which can be hard, given that at times you may not know what is going to happen the next day and may feel pretty powerless to change and accomplish any goal beyond getting to practice, school, and sleep.

Part of setting your own agenda requires that you look at what you want to do beyond college. What are you going to do when your four years of college eligibility ends? You faced a similar situation during your high school career. No one gets to stay a high school student-athlete forever. Likewise, college student-athlete eligibility ends at some point. What can you do today to prepare for that moment?

College is a period of exploration for individuals to choose a career or profession. College students choose a major, take classes, and pursue internships in areas that they are interested in working in once they graduate. As graduation approaches, these individuals spend hours developing resumes, searching for internships, and seeking other experiences that will make them a competitive job applicant in their desired field. Unfortunately, many college students do not take these necessary steps and explore vocational goals prior to graduation. Uncertain of how to even begin selecting or pursuing a career, these students may become quite anxious or despondent. Studies show that many college student-athletes often fall disproportionately into this latter category of students. College student-athletes were also found to engage in less career and educational planning than other students. There are several reasons why student-athletes may be less likely to set career goals and take advantage of career services offered by their schools.

First, some student-athletes, especially at large Division I schools, have a very strong athletic identity and simply perceive that their life role is to be an athlete. These student-athletes completely commit themselves to their sport and often don't even consider other options. Student-athletes who are solely committed to their sport may believe that competing in the sport or something related, such as coaching, is their only viable career option. In this way, sport commitment may limit their career development and limit their willingness to pursue other dreams. As a student-athlete you must be cautious not to limit your options for life after graduation. After all, only a small number of student-athletes will ultimately compete professionally. Thus, when student-athletes' competitive athletic careers are over, they should have alternative occupations in mind. University career centers are valuable resources.

A second factor that often impacts student-athletes' career development is lack of time. Student-athletes usually have more externally imposed time commitments than non-athletes. In addition to their full load of classes, they have workouts, practices, games, travel, and team meetings. Activities related to career development such as visits to the career center, sessions with a career counselor, resume development, and internships may simply not fit into an already hectic schedule. Student-athletes' schedules are rigid and very structured. Coaches and professors place great demands on student-athletes and require them to keep rigid schedules and follow many rules. This externally imposed structure may also inhibit career development in these students, and research suggests that it discourages exploratory behaviors in collegiate athletes, who may feel unprepared to make decisions or explore options independently.

It is important for student-athletes to begin setting goals and thinking about their futures as soon as they begin college. This is not to say that as a freshman you should know exactly what you want to do when you graduate, but rather it means you should start setting goals for yourself and explore different interests and possibilities. First, student-athletes should assess their interests, abilities, personality, and values. Evaluate what you enjoy, what subjects interest you, and what you would look for in an ideal career. Second, explore your

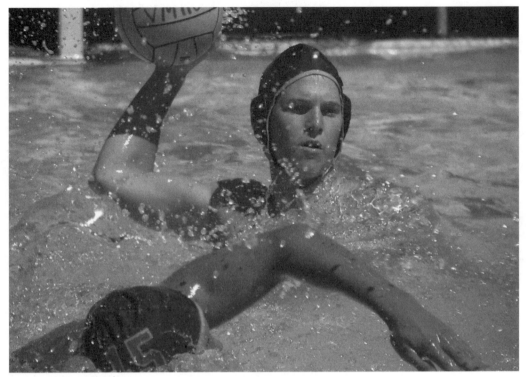

© Chad McDermott/ShutterStock, Inc.

capabilities and develop your skills. Exploration might open a wider range of career options and help you think more broadly about your future. Exploration could mean setting up time to meet with a career planner, learning about different academic majors, or simply keeping an open mind to a class with subject matter you know little about. Next, it is important that you understand both your strengths and weaknesses. Once you identify deficits, locate on-campus services, such as career services or educational support services, that can help you with your career development.

Finally, it is important that you think more broadly about yourself and your future. Create a contingency plan for if you do not go on to play professional sports, and think beyond the immediate. It is helpful to think about and prepare for a wide range of potential life events such as graduation, beginning a job, marriage, moving, or starting a family. Obviously, you cannot plan your entire future while in college, but it is important to explore your options and take advantage of the career development resources available at your school.

THINK ABOUT IT ✓

- ❑ Name something that you were able to do because of your involvement in sports that you would not have been able to do if you were not a student-athlete.

- ❑ What are your long-term goals? How can your experiences as a student-athlete help you achieve these goals?

- ❑ Why is it important for student-athletes to create their own agenda and identify their own goals? How may this help them be successful both in sports and in life?

Caring for Yourself

Typically, student-athletes are very driven to reach their goals. But with goals and agendas set, it is important to remember to take care of yourself and cut yourself some slack. Being a student-athlete can be difficult. Perhaps you are away from home, your family, and friends for the first time and are missing your normal support system. Maybe you have begun to doubt your ability to succeed at college-level work, to build adult relationships, and to adapt to the responsibilities of being a student-athlete. It is certainly normal to feel a little overwhelmed at times. After all, as a student-athlete, you must balance all of the demands of being a college student along with intense athletic demands. This includes the physical demands of playing a sport as well as the time commitment and dedication it takes to participate.

Most student-athletes participate year-round in their sport and often miss holidays, school and summer breaks, as well as classes and school functions. In addition, they may struggle in their performance, experience setbacks, or even play through injury. Finally, student-athletes may have interpersonal troubles, having difficulty interacting with their coach or teammates. All of these things can be very difficult to handle. It is important to understand that no matter how overwhelmed you may feel, there are people out there who can help. You have academic advisers, tutors, trainers, counselors, coaches, and teammates who understand what demands you are facing and are there to help you through the hard times.

As a student-athlete you must recognize when things are hard and when you need help. Second, you must identify what you need to be healthy, feel in control, be happy, and be successful. Finally, you must be willing to ask for help and support when you need it. More often then not, student-athletes struggle to do it all: go to classes, complete their assignments, practice, train, travel to competitions, and maintain their friendships. Inevitably, something has to give.

THINK ABOUT IT

❑ What are some of the resources or services available on campus to student-athletes? Do you take advantage of these resources?

❑ Name one thing that you do to take care of yourself physically, mentally, and emotionally (e.g., make sure to get eight hours of sleep, call your best friend when you feel homesick).

PLUGGED IN TO SPORTS

Student-Athletes and Technology

Take a moment to reflect upon how coaches and players communicate and how advances in technology have changed the way coaches and players communicate. Think back to high school, when you were trying to get recognized by college coaches. Did you create a video of your finest athletic moments to send to recruiters? Did you set up a Web site highlighting your athletic career?

When you were looking at schools, did you research schools online and take virtual tours? Did you e-mail the coach to set up a meeting? Did the coach contact you via phone, e-mail, or text messaging? As the technology and the communication changed, the rules had to adapt as well. For example, the NCAA has rules about how many times a coach can contact a prospective student. The NCAA had to reassess this rule in light of increased use of e-mail and text messaging. Coaches were able to avoid violating the communication with players rule while repeatedly sending text messages to athletes, trying to get them to come to their schools. To protect student-athletes from being pressured by coaches and athletic programs, the NCAA addressed this issue and created a new rule limiting the number of e-mails and texts that a coach or athletic staff member can initiate.

Chapter Summary

Success as a student-athlete requires you to have goals and an agenda that encompass more than your sport and classes. As you confront challenges and other obstacles, your goals and agenda can serve as an anchor that assists in setting a direction and moving forward. You are becoming your own person with many skills and successes. As a student-athlete you can take proactive steps to set your own goals and agenda. Likewise, you can use these same techniques to help prepare for life after sports, and in turn you can write your own agenda for life after college. It is important that student-athletes recognize that not all collegiate athletes go on to play professional sports and that they must begin to explore other career options. Successful student-athletes should go through college with an open mind and take advantage of the wonderful opportunity that they have to receive an education and gain the experience and knowledge needed to pursue a career that is satisfying for them.

Your Thoughts

1. Make a list of qualities that you value in yourself. Are these the qualities that you value in other people? Think about how you might be able to develop those qualities that you value in other people. Can you change your attitude? Why is it important to you to have those values? How can they help you as a student-athlete?

2. Why is it important to have rules for student-athletes? What do you think would happen if there were no rules? Think about the last time you broke the rules. Why did you do it? Were there any consequences? What, if anything, did you take away from the experience?

3. How do you think your parents or guardians have had to adjust to you being in college? What kinds of things have they had to change besides the rules? Do you think it was an easy transition for them or a hard one?

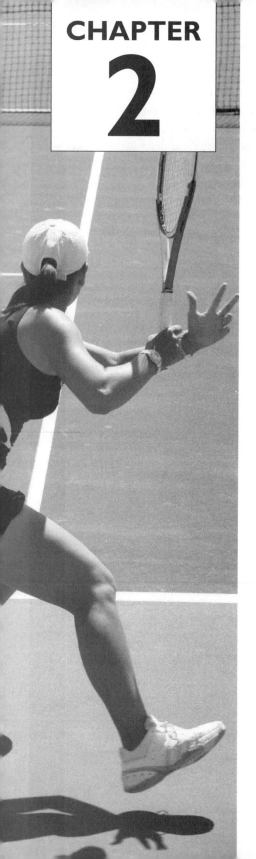

CHAPTER 2

Student-Athlete Challenges

Learning Objectives

After completing this chapter, you will be able to:

- *Identify the eight key challenges that student-athletes face and assess your level of involvement with each of the eight challenges*

- *Understand the three types of stress (physical, psychological, and psychosocial) and be able to classify stress as either chronic or acute*

- *Understand both the physical and mental responses to stress*

- *Explain how stress affects performance both positively and negatively*

- *Identify positive ways to manage and cope with stress*

© Galina Barskaya/ShutterStock, Inc.

Student-Athletes Say:

- I just got back my first paper. The professor scribbled all over it in red pen and gave me a D. I can't believe he didn't like it. I've never gotten a D in my life.

- Practices are so much harder than they were in high school. After the first week of the season, I had shin splints, blisters, and a pulled hamstring. I was in so much pain, I could barely walk.

- The competition in college is pretty tough. I can see why some people think about using steroids or other performance enhancers to get ahead.

- I'm worried about a few girls on my team. They are so obsessed with what they eat and dieting that it's actually scary. They can't possibly be eating enough to stay healthy and play their best.

- With practices and games all week and tournaments on the weekends, it doesn't leave much time for socializing, much less partying. Other kids on my hall go out and come home late, most of them drunk. Sometimes I'm a little jealous that they can get away with that kind of behavior and I can't.

- I have morning workouts before class, practice after class, weekend practices and games, and a boyfriend giving me a hard time. It is hard and stressful not having time to spend with him.

- A friend of mine played basketball at a big state school and one of his teammates was accused of shaving points. I couldn't even imagine not being able to trust your own teammate. My teammates are like my family.

You're probably doing all of the things that are expected of you: going to practice, lifting, competing, trying to eat well, working with your coaches, going to classes, spending time on course assignments, studying for tests, writing papers, developing friendships, going to parties, and maybe even maintaining some responsibilities at home. You are doing a lot.

As a student-athlete you are pulled in a number of different directions by people, all of whom have your best interest at heart but may not share common goals for you. For your professors, your performance in the classroom is the highest priority. How you complete the course assignments, readings, and projects are what they care the most about. They may not even know (or care) that you are a student-athlete. Your coach expects your full participation and total commitment to your sport and team. From your coach's point of view, your athletic performance needs to be your single highest priority in life. Your parents, guardians, and family members may give you mixed messages about what needs to be your priority: classes and/or athletics. Your school, teammates, and friends all want to give you advice on what to do and how you should spend your time.

Student-athletes are special people. On campus you are a member of the most easily identifiable group of individuals by faculty, students, parents, community members, the administration, the board of trustees, alumni, and media. You are known by people you have never met. At times, you are at the mercy of other people's decisions and actions. And all you want is to be able to pursue the goal of achieving academic success and competitive athletic performance at the college level.

Your college student-athlete experience is different from your athletic experience in the previous twelve years of school. In college you have a lot more freedom to live the way you want, and with that freedom, you have greater responsibilities. Unless you are living at home while attending school, the college student-athlete experience is one in which you transition from a period of dependence (on your parents, guardians, or extended family) to independence. As you move from the known to the unknown, the list of stressors you may experience is rather startling. Box 2.1 lists some of the more common stressors that college students face as well as some additional ones that college student-athletes face. These are only examples.

STUDENT REFLECTION

Box 2.1. What Are Your Sources of Stress?

Here is a list of sources of stress for all college students (including student-athletes) and some additional sources of college student-athlete stress (**). Can you list other sources of stress in your life as a college student-athlete?

Roommate dynamics	Trying to fit in and feel accepted by people
Picking a major	Working
Exams, papers, and projects	Practice schedule (**)
Financial aid and school loans	Conditioning (**)
Budgeting your money	Coaches (**)
Freedom to stay up and get up when when you want	Competition (**)
Making friends	Athletic performance (**)
Exploring sexuality	
Meeting a special person you want to spend time with	
Family responsibilities	

Balancing academics and college life is hard enough. Adding athletics to the mix results in your life becoming a juggling act extraordinaire. In the process of meeting everyone else's needs and demands, your needs and time can very quickly be squeezed with no time left for you. In the end everything can suffer. You end up feeling frustrated over the inadequacy of your time and effort to meet the demands.

Last fall, the head of the department decided to change the name of a course I was enrolled in. In order to change the course name so it would show up correctly on everyone's transcripts, my adviser had to drop everyone from the class and re-enroll them into the new course. She was planning on doing this over the course of a few days between classes and her appointments with students. When she dropped all of the students from the class, I was not added to the new class roster for a couple of days. In the meantime, I had a big lacrosse game coming up in Maryland. I was on my way to board the team bus for the trip, and our compliance officer called me and said that I was ineligible because I was below the mandatory twelve-credit limit. I knew I had enrolled for twelve credits, but I was completely unaware that my name was not yet added to the new course roster. Twenty minutes before the bus was scheduled to leave, I had to run across campus to my adviser's office and ask her to add me to the roster of the new course immediately. She said she would be getting to it in a few days and not to worry, but she didn't understand that she had to do it NOW, otherwise I would not be allowed to board the bus to the airport! She obviously didn't know the rule about the twelve-credit limit since I was the only student-athlete she was advising. After a stressful hour, I was finally eligible again, and able to travel with my team.

Being a college student-athlete is rewarding, but it is not easy. In this chapter you will prepare to face the challenges of being a successful college student-athlete. You will gain an awareness of the challenges and the accompanying stress. You'll be introduced to strategies that student-athletes use to cope with and manage the challenges and stress.

Understanding Student-Athlete Challenges

Challenges test your abilities. Challenges push you to learn using all of your abilities (intelligence) even when you are not sure of yourself. In the process, you may feel awkward and uncomfortable. At the top of your list of challenges is peak performance as both a student and an athlete. Ranking right next to peak performance is making good decisions, and this book is designed to help you make good decisions about your health and behavior.

The college years are times of achievement and success as well as much anxiety and soul searching. As a competent and caring individual, you need to make good decisions and healthy choices in pursuing your dreams. You possess many positive assets and protective qualities that lead to you being a competent, resilient, and caring individual. You have already used these traits to make many good decisions about your health and behavior.

THINK ABOUT IT ✔

❑ What expectations do coaches have of you? What is expected of you from your professors? How are these expectations similar? Different?

❑ How are challenges different between teams and genders?

While pursuing your goals as a student-athlete, you will face a lot of challenges and stress. But don't worry; you will not face them alone. You will get help, support, and guidance from parents, guardians, coaches, professors, athletic directors, and peers. Even with support resources available, not all college student-athletes are successful. Some run into academic challenges, and the demands of getting a college degree take precedence over the athletics. For others, the physical demands of practice and competition and lack of proper sleep at times undermine the best intentions to attend class and study. Physical injuries prevent full athletic participation. Most distressing is that sometimes the demands of classes and athletic dreams collide in unhealthy choices involving drugs, alcohol, violence, and sex. Colleges and universities have programs to address your academic needs and challenges. For example, most schools have a learning support and academic development center offering academic support, mentoring, and learning aids. Your school may be less prepared to help you deal with the stress and challenges of pursuing your academic and athletic dreams. It really comes back to you to figure out how best to deal with the challenges—to you making the best choices for yourself. Discussed in this chapter is how to prepare for the challenges of being a college student-athlete.

Facing the Challenges

Eight Student-Athlete Challenges

As a student-athlete you are often held to high standards, your performance is scrutinized, you are highly visible on campus, and you are often viewed as a role model. These factors place added pressure and stress on student-athletes, and make it even more critical that student-athletes monitor their behavior and make good, healthy decisions. Student-athletes must monitor everything from the foods they eat, to the language they use, to their decisions whether or not to use drugs, and making good, healthy decisions all the time is not always easy.

People do not always handle high levels of stress in healthy ways. For example, one student-athlete who is stressed over an exam may find that smoking a cigarette relieves some tension. Another student may choose to go out and get drunk on a Friday night to unwind after an especially hard week. Another might smoke marijuana when stressed, while someone else might grab a tub of ice cream after a bad day. Unfortunately, these behaviors can become problematic as people use these coping mechanisms to mask their stress rather than resolve the stressful situations. Over time, people can fall into patterns of poor behavior.

For college student-athletes the concern is with eight student-athlete challenges. Given the pressure-cooker reality of college student-athletes it is important for you to know the eight challenges and pay attention to them. The goal is to prevent health problems and problem behaviors that might hinder your ability to achieve academic success and competitive athletic performance. Each one of the challenges is discussed in this text. The eight challenges are:

- Academics
- Pain and injury
- Nutrition
- Performance enhancers
- Alcohol
- Tobacco, marijuana, and other drugs
- Sex and relationships
- Gambling and money

These challenges are all probably very familiar to you. And depending on your personal life, your knowledge and involvement with each one will vary. For example, you may share with friends and teammates some similarities and common experiences related to a couple of the challenges. With other challenges your experience is personal and private. It is important to recognize and validate the good decisions you are already making about your health each day. At the same time, you need to be prepared with tools and skills to help you better meet the challenges you face.

Involvement with the Challenges

When do unhealthy choices and decisions lead to problem behavior? No one is perfect and makes healthy decisions all the time. It is important to understand when your choices are becoming a problem in your life or affecting your health, relationships, performance, and well-being. Looking at your involvement with the challenges is a good place to start to gain an awareness of their role in your life.

There are five levels of involvement. They range from awareness of a challenge but with no involvement or abstinence to high involvement with perhaps negative personal outcomes such as an addiction with physiological and psychological dependence. The levels of involvement reflect a person's knowledge, attitude, and behavior in relation to the challenge. The levels of involvement can fluctuate, reflecting daily changes as well as long-term patterns and behaviors.

Likewise, differences are expected based on the particular challenge. For example, it is expected that everyone would have a high level of involvement related to academics and nutrition, while the pain and injury involvement would reflect your current physical conditioning and health, which is subject to change over the course of a season. If you were injury and pain free, it is expected you would report low involvement in those challenges. Likewise, the challenges related to substances (e.g., alcohol, tobacco, marijuana) will vary according to individual use. The rating of involvement is judgment free. It is neither positive nor negative but rather reflects your current state as you define it.

Another thing to consider when thinking about the challenges is whether your involvement with the challenge adds any value to your life or your health. In other words, when you talk about the role of the challenge in your life, are you proud of how you address the challenge? For example, when you talk with your coaches and family, can you talk about being highly involved with your academics (e.g., completing assignments, doing well on exams, and attending class), and are they proud and happy for you in your success? Likewise, most people would see not being involved with gambling as adding value to your experience. Managing all of the challenges well can enhance your performance on the field and in the classroom and add value to your agenda as a college student-athlete. Below are the levels of involvement. Use the levels to evaluate the degree to which you engage in each of the challenges.

1. **Never: No Involvement/Abstinence**—No daily contact, use, or behavior related to the challenge. You may be aware of the challenge (e.g., alcohol, marijuana, pain, gambling) but it is not part of your life.

2. **Hardly Ever: Low Involvement/Experimentation**—Infrequent contact, use, or behavior related to the challenge (e.g., tried cigarettes or alcohol once or twice). You have some knowledge of possible consequences and outcomes related to the challenge.

3. **Sometimes: Limited Involvement/Social or Recreational Use**—Occasional contact, use, or behavior related to the challenge (e.g., weekly use of social drinking, sleep aids, cybersex). You have knowledge and experience with consequences and outcomes related to the challenge.

4. **Often: Moderate Involvement/Daily**—Daily contact, use, or behavior related to the challenge. You have knowledge and experience with consequences and outcomes related to the challenge (e.g., pain medication use for injury pain relief, smoking marijuana to relax).

5. **Almost Always: High Involvement/Frequent Daily Use**—Frequent daily contact, use, or behavior related to the challenge. You have knowledge and experience with consequences and outcomes related to the challenge (e.g., completing class assignments, Internet gambling, dietary supplements).

As you go forward in this book it is helpful to think about your involvement with each of the challenges as a way to promote your health and success as a student-athlete. Complete the form in Box 2.2 to get a quick assessment of your current levels of involvement. Check (✓) the box that corresponds to your level of involvement (1, 2, 3, 4, 5). In the final columns, check (✓) if this challenge or how you engage with it is adding value to your life (+), neutral in your life (o),

Box 2.2. **Student-Athlete Challenges**

Directions: Evaluate each statement on a scale of 1 to 5, from 1 being "never" to 5 being "almost always." For each statement evaluate if your behavior adds value to (+), is neutral (0), or decreases value (−) of your student-athlete success in regard to your classes and sport.

Statement	Never				Almost Always	Value Added		
	1	2	3	4	5	+	0	−
Academics	❑	❑	❑	❑	❑	❑	❑	❑
Pain and injury	❑	❑	❑	❑	❑	❑	❑	❑
Nutrition	❑	❑	❑	❑	❑	❑	❑	❑
Performance enhancers	❑	❑	❑	❑	❑	❑	❑	❑
Alcohol	❑	❑	❑	❑	❑	❑	❑	❑
Tobacco, marijuana, and other drugs	❑	❑	❑	❑	❑	❑	❑	❑
Sex and relationships	❑	❑	❑	❑	❑	❑	❑	❑
Gambling and money	❑	❑	❑	❑	❑	❑	❑	❑

or a distraction that actually causes you to lose personal value, time, and energy or causes you stress (−). For example, you might play online poker about once a week. You've never bet or lost more than $10. You usually play a few hands when you are procrastinating and don't feel like writing a paper for class. Your level of involvement is a 3. Your gambling is not adding value to your life—in fact, it is distracting you from completing your homework, therefore you rate that it has a negative (−) value added.

As you complete the quick assessment in Box 2.2, do you see any patterns? Many student-athletes' answers are a mix, evaluating themselves as a 4 or 5 on some challenges, a 1 or 2 on others, and as a 3 on the remainder. What is your pattern?

Challenges cause stress in your life. Often we think of stress as an externally imposing aspect of our lives that threatens or makes a demand on our minds and bodies. But for most of us, stress usually results from an internal state of emotional tension that occurs in response to the various demands or challenges of living. Most current definitions state that stress is the mental and physical response of our bodies to the challenges in our lives. It is also known that we make choices about how we deal with stress. As a student-athlete you can make those choices. To help you understand the ways you might cope with and manage your stress, the next section explores how you react to stress and describes stress-management strategies.

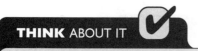

THINK ABOUT IT

- ❑ Discuss how a challenge can be both positive and negative.
- ❑ Are all challenges created equal? Are some more important than others? What is the most difficult challenge that you face as a student-athlete?

Challenges and Stress

Physical Response to Stress

When people experience stress, they respond in remarkably similar and predictable ways. For example, when surprised by a sudden stressor, such as a car swerving into their lane of traffic, most people react by swerving to avoid the crash. This automatic reaction is known as the stress response or the physiological and psychological response to positive or negative events that are disruptive, unexpected, or stimulating. Physiologically, when a person encounters stress, the adrenal glands immediately respond. The glands that control this reaction are located on top of the kidneys and secrete adrenaline and other hormones into the bloodstream. As a result, the heart speeds up, breathing rate increases, blood pressure elevates, and the flow of blood to the muscles increases with a rapid release of blood sugars into the bloodstream. This sudden burst of energy and strength is believed to provide the extra edge that has helped generations of humans survive during adversity, known as the fight-or-flight response. A physiological reaction is believed to be one of the most basic and innate survival instincts. Our bodies go into an alert mode and prepare to either fight or escape. The natural, physiological response to stress follows a distinct pattern. The human body moves through three stages when confronted with these stressors (see Figure 2.1).

During the alarm stage, involuntary changes controlled by the hormonal and nervous systems trigger the fight-or-flight response. For example, you may realize that you are an hour late for practice because you have forgotten that the coach wanted the team to come an hour early. You may begin to experience feelings of fear, panic, anxiety, anger, depression, and restlessness.

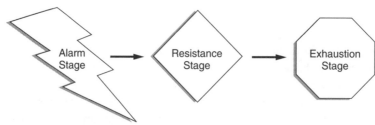

Figure 2.1 Three Phases of Stress

Resistance, the second stage, is when the body attempts to reestablish its equilibrium or internal balance. When the body experiences the alarm stage for a prolonged amount of time, it naturally goes into survival mode. The body will resist or attempt to resolve the problem and reduce the intensity of the response to a more manageable level. During this phase, you might take steps to calm yourself down and relieve the stress on your body. For instance, you may deny the situation or withdraw and isolate yourself from others, including ignoring your emotions. For example, referring to the scenario above, you may decide to pretend that you are sick and skip practice rather than showing up late to practice and facing the consequences of running extra laps.

Of course, the longer your body is under stress and out of balance, the more negative the impact. If your body experiences a prolonged lack of control and balance, an exhaustion stage occurs, causing your stress-management resources to collapse and the stress-producing hormones, such as adrenaline, to rise. During this stage, your body begins to develop chronic and serious illnesses. Long-term exposure to a stressor or exposure to multiple stressors at the same time often results in overloading your system. For instance, if the player from the example above continues to lie about missing practice, he or she may feel extreme guilt that could lead to an anxiety disorder.

Research on these three stages has indicated that there is a strong connection between continuous exposure to a high level of stress and an increased risk for disease. In fact, stress is also

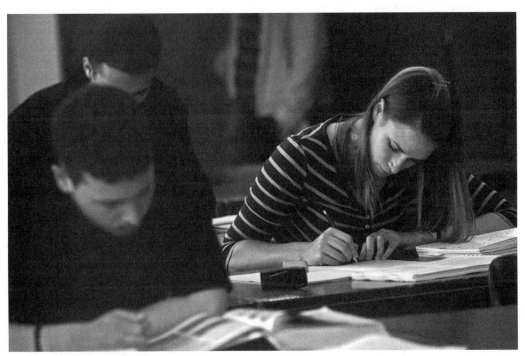

© PhotoCreate/ShutterStock, Inc.

described generically as a "disease of prolonged arousal" that often leads to other negative health effects. Nearly all systems of the body can become potential targets of this assault, and the long-term effects may be devastating. Almost every system in your body can be damaged by stress. For example, prolonged stress can cause suppression of the reproduction system, as illustrated by the cessation of menstruation in women, impotency in men, and loss of libido (sexual drive) in both. Stress also jeopardizes the respiratory system because it can trigger changes in the lungs and increase the symptoms of asthma, bronchitis, and other respiratory conditions. Stress weakens the skeletal system by suspending tissue repair, which in turn causes decalcification of the bones, osteoporosis, and susceptibility to fractures. Inhibition of immune and inflammatory systems makes you more susceptible to colds and flu. When the immune system is vulnerable, it can intensify the possibility of developing some diseases and/or chronic conditions such as cancer, AIDS, arthritis, and diabetes. There are also some types of chronic stress that can contribute to anxiety, depression, and/or mental disorders. Chronic or persistent stress can occur when the stressors of life prove to be unrelenting, as they may be during the transition from high school to college or the juggling of school work and your sport.

It is important to remember that physical symptoms may have purely physiological causes. You should have a medical doctor eliminate the possibility of such physical problems before you proceed on the assumption that your symptoms are completely stress related. As you gain more control and your balance is reestablished, you can begin to recover from the stressors causing issues in your life.

Mental Response to Stress

Stressors manifest in all shapes, sizes, and degrees of intensity. Many scholars concur that it is not the circumstance that is stressful but the perception or interpretation of the circumstance that elicits stress. If the perception is negative, it can become both a mental and physical liability. With any stressful event we encounter, our perceptions can become distorted and magnified entirely out of proportion to their seriousness. This is referred to as cognitive distortion because it can make minor incidents seem gigantic.

The working of the human mind is extremely complex, something that we are only beginning to comprehend. Negative perceptions are often the result of low self-esteem. They also perpetuate it by suppressing feelings of self-worth and self-acceptance. Have you ever gotten all worked up about something you thought was happening only to find that your perceptions were totally wrong or that a communication problem had caused a misinterpretation of events? It is a human behavior to misinterpret communication, and most often people get upset not by realities but by their skewed perceptions. For example, suppose you found out that everybody except you was invited to a party. It is natural to wonder why you did not receive an invitation and if the reason you did not get invited is because someone dislikes you, or perhaps you offended someone. Regardless of your concerns, neither of these realities may be true and the situation may have absolutely nothing to do with your being liked or disliked. Perhaps you were sent an invitation but it did not reach you in time. Or maybe the host of the party invited your teammate and assumed that she or he would mention going to the party to you. This type of thinking is called self-talk.

For most people, almost every minute of their conscious life involves engaging in self-talk. This is your internal thought language, including sentences with which you describe and interpret the world. Most peoples' self-talk is accurate and they are usually in touch with reality. Psychologist Albert Ellis developed a system to attack irrational ideas or beliefs and replace them with realistic statements. He called this system Rational Emotive Behavior Therapy and introduced it first in *A Guide to Rational Living* with co-author Robert Harper in 1961. Ellis's basic theory is that emotions have nothing to do with actual events, and in between the events and the emotions is realistic or unrealistic self-talk. In fact, it is self-talk that produces your emotions. Your own thoughts, directed and controlled by you, are what create anxiety, anger, and depression. If your self-talk is irrational and untrue, then you experience stress and emotional disturbance; however, if your self-talk is up-lifting and positive, it might be a source of motivation or positive reinforcement. An example of ir-rational self-talk may include, "If I do not make every basket, I do not deserve to be on the team." Instead, student-athletes should use positive self-talk, telling themselves that even if they do not make the team, they had to opportunity to meet new people and experiences.

Furthermore, irrational ideas can be thought of as outright misperceptions, such as, "If we lose our first game, the entire season is over." In addition, a player can learn to recognize neg-ative perfectionism (which Ellis calls "shoulds, oughts, and musts") in such self-talk as, "I must play my best or I will let my friends and family down." Instead, student-athletes can reflect on the fact that their friends and family will love them no matter how they play.

Performance and Stress

Stress and strain are associated with sports as well as with most daily activities. As with anything, some stress is good, but too much can be unhealthy. The four main types of stress people gen-erally physically experience are called hypostress, eustress, hyperstress, and distress (Figure 2.2).

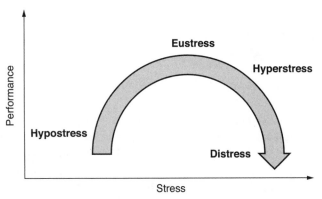

Figure 2.2 Human Function Curve: Effects of Stress on Performance

First, hypostress occurs when an individual is bored or unchallenged, or when a person doesn't have enough stress in her life. People who feel hypostress may be restless or uninspired. For example, during the season a female cross-country runner is accustomed to excelling and running at her peak speed for three miles each day, with a time around nineteen minutes. When the season ends, she decides to run three miles every day with her younger sister to stay in shape; spending approximately twenty-five minutes for each running session. By the time the season starts again, the cross-country runner can no longer run a three-mile course in nineteen minutes—instead, it takes her twenty-one minutes. In these scenarios, the athlete fails to perform at an optimum level due to an absence of stress, loss of motivation, and elimination of competition; thus, when experiencing hypostress, a little added stress may have a positive effect.

Generally, positive stress, or stress that presents the opportunity for personal growth and satisfaction, is called eustress. For instance, examples of eustress in daily life include starting school, beginning a career, developing new friendships, and learning a new physical skill. How does this relate to performance? For instance, if the cross-country runner from the example above ran each day with a friend at her same speed or a little faster rather than running slower with her little sister, she is more likely to perform at the same level or improve for her upcoming season. An athlete's body needs stress to stimulate the body's stress response, which triggers it to adapt and perform better. Stress presents a challenge that causes an athlete's abilities to improve; thus, athletes need many levels of stress to perform their best.

Unlike eustress, hyperstress occurs when an individual is pushed beyond a level that he or she can handle. Hyperstress results from being overloaded or overworked. When someone is hyperstressed, little events can trigger a strong emotional response. For example, athletes training during their off season may be mentally and physically overworked and prone to injury or burnout by the pre-season.

The last type of stress is distress. Distress, a negative stress, is caused by those events that result in disabling stress and strain. For instance, examples of negative distress can include financial problems, the death of a loved one, academic difficulties, the breakup of a relationship, or an injury that puts you out of play.

THINK ABOUT IT

❑ Think of the last time you were in a stressful or uncomfortable situation. How did your body physically react?

❑ Sometimes we create added stress for ourselves by overthinking things, psyching ourselves out, or having negative self-talk. Give an example of how negative thoughts or mental stress can prevent an athlete from being successful.

❑ Describe a time when you performed at your best. What stressors were present that helped you rise to your maximum potential?

Dealing with Stress

Coping with and Managing Stress

Many student-athletes have discovered positive strategies and methods for stress management including the physical, social, environmental, and psychological aspects of their stress. For example, one of the best ways to mobilizing yourself to cope with a difficult situation is to understand how and why it makes you anxious. What particular aspects of the situation will be most difficult to manage? What might be your worst fears about the outcomes? At which points do you feel most out of control of your emotions? The answers to these questions may not always be clear, particularly if you face complex situations. However, the more you understand about the situations you may be facing, the easier it will be to cope. How would you handle this problematic situation? Your coach is angry because you were late for practice and tells you that you will not be starting for the next conference game as a consequence of your continued tardiness. Our autonomic nervous system produces symptoms such as tightness in the stomach, sweating, and palpitations. How you interpret the incident and imagine how it will affect your future will affect your emotions and feelings of self-worth. For example, if you say to yourself, "I have lost my spot on the team," you are stating a prediction. Instead, you may want to reflect inwardly and think, "I'm too disorganized and irresponsible to continue to be a starter." An interpretation of the event could include thinking, "I know he wants me to sit the bench or wants me off the team," and your physiological response will probably include sweating and/or a knot in your stomach. Noticing your physical reactions, you might then think, "I can't do this anymore; I can't handle the pressures of school and being an athlete." These negative self-statements in turn can increase the physiological symptoms and the tendency to make poor decisions. A vicious cycle of negative thoughts to physical reactions and behavioral choices can lead toward more negative thoughts and a continued unbroken state of chronic stress. Your thoughts do not have to intensify fear; instead, they can act as tranquilizers for a tense stomach, including calming you and pushing you away from panic. Stress-coping thoughts tell your body there is no need for arousal; it can relax. In the middle of any stressful situation, you can begin saying to yourself a series of fear-conquering statements such as, "Stay calm . . . you can earn your spot back . . . relax . . . I will prove myself to the coach." The more attention you give to your coping monologue, the quicker it will give relief from physiological arousal.

Below are a number of strategies that student-athletes report using to deal with their stress. Review the list. Most strategies can be adapted to a variety of situations. Later in the book we will discuss effective strategies to deal with specific challenges that you face as a student-athlete.

- *Take a break*—Schedule several short breaks throughout the day to help minimize your stress. Get up and stretch, go for a walk, or call a friend. When you return to your work, you will work more efficiently.

- *Minimize interruptions*—When you have something important to get done, make sure to block off a period of time when you can work without being disturbed or distracted. Put your phone on voicemail, shut your door, or go someplace to work where no one can find you.

- *Practice daily relaxation exercises*—Effective daily relaxation exercises include deep breathing, progressive muscle relaxation (PMR), and visualization.

- *Think positively and learn to control worry*—Instead of focusing on negative thoughts, focus on the positive aspects in your life and tell yourself at least one positive thought each day. Do not waste your time worrying about things you cannot change or always planning for the worst.

- *Learn to say no*—Do not feel guilty when you have to tell others "no." If you accept additional projects or work for others when you are busy, it will only lead to additional stress.

- *Put stressful situations in perspective*—Will it matter a month from now? What about a year from now?

- *Get enough sleep*—Most people need between six and nine hours, but many people lose sleep when they are under stress to finish more work.

Resiliency

You know that your life is stressful. And this is not good or bad but rather a reality of being a student-athlete. Knowing this fact allows you to anticipate and prepare for stressful days, examinations, classes, practices, and competitions. You will not be able to avoid stress, but perhaps you can be better prepared when the day-to-day hassles, stresses you know about, as well as those that are surprises cluster together to catch you off guard. In other words, you want to build your resiliency—your ability to bounce back from stress and adversity.

Developing competencies, or resiliency skills, is a key factor in successfully responding to life's stresses and adversities. It *is* possible to be hurt and rebound at the same time. Resilient individuals refrain from blaming themselves for what has gone wrong. Through a process called "adaptive distancing" they can draw boundaries between the problem and themselves. "My situation is troubled, but I am not my situation." They maintain their independence and are often drawn to spending time with healthier peers and families.

Ongoing research indicates that those who are resilient take responsibility for what goes right in their lives. They cultivate insight, they are able to be honest, and they take charge of problems. They have good decision-making and planning skills, a healthy sense of humor, and a sense of hope about the future. They know how to ask for help and support when they need it, and how to cultivate relationships that provide that.

THINK ABOUT IT ✔

- ❏ People often describe their reaction to stress using metaphors (e.g., "I have a splitting headache," "My stomach was in a knot," "I am in a fog."). What metaphors can you think of to describe your reaction to stress (physical or mental)?
- ❏ Reflect on how self-talk has affected your mental state at practice or in competition.
- ❏ Think of a time you perceived a situation one way and then found out that your interpretation was inaccurate or exaggerated. How did you react? What could you have done differently?

Reframing is at the heart of resilience. It is a way of shifting the focus to the cup being half-full instead of half-empty. Going back to an incident, finding the strengths, and building self-esteem from the achievement are what build resilience. Instead of seeing oneself as a "helpless victim" one can reframe an experience to see oneself as a "victor." This is a critical step in developing resilience: shifting from a "deficit model" to a "competence model."

The two perspectives speak for themselves: "look at how horrible your life has been and how you've been victimized" or "look at how you managed to survive and thrive in spite of it." Sometimes it's easier to be the victim; it removes the obligation to change. It is also possible to emerge from difficult situations with dignity and strength and lead a healthy and gratifying life.

A resilient student-athlete is one who is:

1. *Positive*—Sees life as challenging, dynamic, and filled with opportunities. "I will do this."

2. *Focused*—Determines where he or she is headed and sticks to that goal so that barriers do not block his or her way. "What is it?"

3. *Flexible*—Open to different possibilities when faced with uncertainty. "I am able to do this."

4. *Organized*—Develops structured approaches to be able to manage the unknown. "What do I need to do?"

5. *Proactive*—Looks ahead, actively engages change, and works with it. "I got through it. What is next?"

Chapter Summary

As a student-athlete, you will face eight challenges as you progress in your athletic and academic career. The challenges are sources of stress and, depending on the particular challenges as well as the level of involvement, can have a positive or a negative impact on you.

PLUGGED IN TO SPORTS

Student-Athletes and Technology

Technology is supposed to make our life easier, right? Unfortunately, that's not always the case. Ever experience information overload? Think about a normal day and how you are surrounded with high-tech gizmos and gadgets. You use technologies so frequently that you probably do not even realize the actual amount of time you spend using them. For example, on a typical day you may wake up to a digital alarm clock, turn on the radio or television, check your e-mail and/or favorite Web sites, all before going to class. During your commute to class, you text message a classmate by using your cell phone. As you walk across campus, you listen to your favorite morning radio show on your MP3 player. Once in class, you take notes on a laptop or use a lull in class lecture to instant message (IM) a friend, play a quick game of solitaire, or visit MySpace.com.

As technology has changed people have become more and more interconnected. We have become a culture on the move and on the phone. If you stop and look at the people around you, you will notice many people walking down the street, on the bus, and in their cars constantly trying to stay connected through devices such as cell phones, laptops, and BlackBerries. The use of cell phones and other communication technologies has become so excessive that many businesses now have signs asking that people kindly turn off their cell phones.

While communication has become faster and in some ways easier, there is a fear that we have become too accessible, distracted, and even impersonal. A constant stream of messages, e-mails, and calls can actually be frustrating as it becomes hard to decipher what communication is important. Student-athletes need to be careful with the overuse of cell phones and know when to turn them off and escape from constant communication.

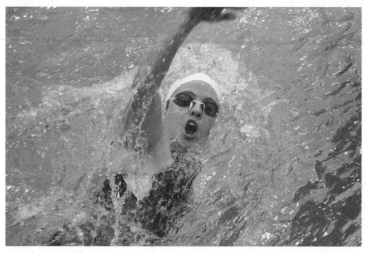

©Erik Patton/ShutterStock, Inc.

We react to stress in specific ways. The stress response is the physiological and psychological response to positive or negative events that can be disruptive, unexpected, or stimulating. The fight-or-flight response is a physiological response to a perceived and anticipated threat. The fight-or-flight response causes the heart to race, breathing becomes labored, muscles are tense, the body sweats, and blood flow is constricted to the extremities and digestive organs and increases to the major muscles in the brain. There are typical stages of stress responses that the body goes through to adapt to present stressors: alarm, resistance, and exhaustion.

Stressors can either positively or negatively affect sports or academic performance. Undue stress for extended periods of time can compromise the immune system. Although increasing evidence links disease susceptibility to stress, much of this research is controversial. Stress has been linked to numerous health problems including high blood pressure, headaches, backaches, fatigue, and depression. All stimuli received by the brain are processed through interpretation and classified as negative, neutral, or positive; this process is called perception. Interpretation that is exaggerated is referred to as cognitive distortion.

One key skill area of successful student-athletes is the ability to deal with stress. You need to recognize the signs of stress and learn to reduce and cope with multiple stressors, such as balancing school work with athletic practice and games. Managing stress begins with learning simple coping mechanisms, assessing stressors, changing responses, and learning to cope. It is important to find out what works best for you; however, probably some combination of managing emotional responses, taking mental or physical action, learning time management, or using alternative stress management techniques may assist in your quest to cope with stress better. Finally, you want to not only deal with stress but to be resilient facing the challenges and stress you know you will encounter as a student-athlete.

Your Thoughts

1. Does knowing about the eight student-athlete challenges help you face them? Would it be better to perhaps not talk about them and just try the best you can to avoid problems?

2. Stress knows no gender boundaries. Men and women both experience stress. We know that effective stress management must address issues related to social, emotional, mental, physical, and spiritual well-being. Do you believe men and women approach stress in their lives differently? Identify among your friends (both women and men) similarities and differences in how they manage stress.

3. We deal with stress differently at different times in our lives. How did you deal with stress in high school? How has that changed now that you are a university student? Do you think that you deal with stress better or worse now than you did when you were in high school?

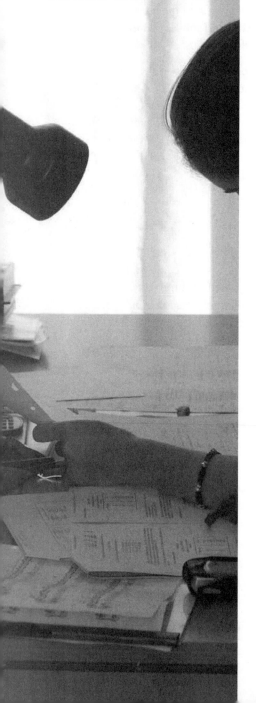

CHAPTER 3

Challenge #1: Academics

Learning Objectives

After completing this chapter, you will be able to:

- *Understand the differences between high school and college and obtain skills to help you with the transition*

- *Be a proactive learner by building relationships with professors and understanding policies and procedures*

- *Manage your time by keeping a calendar, making to-do lists, prioritizing tasks, and mapping out your day*

- *Apply skills for taking notes, writing papers, and preparing for and taking tests*

© Jerome Scholler/ShutterStock, Inc.

Student-Athletes Say:

- I take so many notes in class my hand hurts. I don't know if I will ever be able to study and remember everything the professors say.

- The quiz had twenty-five multiple-choice questions and a short essay. I can't imagine what a test will be.

- I thought I wrote a decent paper, but the professor wrote all over it and told me to try again.

- Last semester, I was studying, practicing hard, and trying to do too much at once. I was barely sleeping four hours a night and wasn't eating very well. I ended up getting really sick after finals week.

- During my junior year in college, I finally mastered the art of effective time management. I ran track, and I learned to set aside time in the morning before practice to do school work so that after practice or meets when I was tired, I could just relax and have some time for myself.

- Last year, a friend of mine played baseball for a big school. After his first year, he had a 1.76 GPA and he wasn't allowed to continue playing baseball. He even lost his scholarship. Seeing what he went through, I knew I had to get off to a good start academically. I don't want anything to jeopardize my eligibility.

Many years ago, when student-athletes arrived on campus their performance in the classroom was not a priority. Often it was left to them to "sink or swim" in their classes. If they disappeared, dropped out, or were allowed to slide through, it really did not matter as long as they played their sport. And although a team might miss them if they "disappeared," there was always another student coming along to fill the void they left behind. Sadly, many of these early student-athletes never got an education, a degree, or a start toward a meaningful and productive career.

Today success in the classroom is equal in importance to success on the playing field. Being academically eligible is a requirement for college student-athletes. The first challenge for college student-athletes is academics. Large classes, class projects, and increased amounts of writing and reading are issues faced by every new college student including new college student-athletes. Even students who have continuously excelled in the classroom or took advanced placement courses in high school can have difficulty transitioning to the college learning environment. Different skills are needed to succeed in college than in high school, junior college, or two-year colleges. The demands are greater and there is a greater need for self-discipline in your studies. Many student-athletes identify their number-one fear as "flunking out" but may not be familiar with the academic (learning) skills they need to navigate their courses successfully. Many do not realize the level of work expected of them at college.

This chapter focuses on the learning skills you need to meet the academic challenges. Schools do care about you getting an education, learning, completing a degree, and developing a realistic and meaningful career plan. To get started, complete the Student-Athlete Challenge # 1: Academics Self-Assessment in Box 3.1. Think about how you are as a student. What is your pattern and style? What are your attitude and behavior in class? How can your academics add value to your success as a student-athlete?

Box 3.1. Student-Athlete Challenge #1 *Academics Self-Assessment*

Directions: Evaluate each statement on a scale of 1 to 5, from 1 being "never" to 5 being "almost always." For each statement evaluate if your behavior adds value (+), is neutral (0), or decreases value (−) of your student-athlete success in regard to your classes and sport.

Statement	Never				Almost Always	Value Added		
	1	2	3	4	5	+	0	−
1. I keep my materials for classes organized in a binder or organizer.	❏	❏	❏	❏	❏	❏	❏	❏
2. I use a day planner to manage my time and plan my day.	❏	❏	❏	❏	❏	❏	❏	❏
3. I visit my professor or teaching assistant during office hours.	❏	❏	❏	❏	❏	❏	❏	❏
4. I take thorough notes during class.	❏	❏	❏	❏	❏	❏	❏	❏
5. I feel prepared and confident when I take tests.	❏	❏	❏	❏	❏	❏	❏	❏
6. I go to the academic support center on campus.	❏	❏	❏	❏	❏	❏	❏	❏
7. I do my assigned readings for class.	❏	❏	❏	❏	❏	❏	❏	❏
8. I am comfortable speaking in class and asking or answering questions.	❏	❏	❏	❏	❏	❏	❏	❏
9. I study for exams by cramming the night before.	❏	❏	❏	❏	❏	❏	❏	❏
10. I e-mail my instructors to let them know that I will be out of town for a game or meet.	❏	❏	❏	❏	❏	❏	❏	❏
11. I have used being an athlete as an excuse to get an extension on a project or get out of an academic responsibility.	❏	❏	❏	❏	❏	❏	❏	❏
12. I visit the writing center for extra help when I have a challenging paper to write.	❏	❏	❏	❏	❏	❏	❏	❏

Every day is a school day when you are in college. And each professor sees his or her class as the most important. It is up you to meet the demands of not just one professor but every professor you have each term. Professors expect and require you to work before, during, and after class. And to be eligible to play, you need to meet this challenge.

> From the first minute of class the professor was writing on the board and flipping through a PowerPoint presentation. He gave out the class Web site and told us to download the lecture notes and read the class blog. He fired off a steady stream of ideas, dates, and details. I was taken back. I just listened for several minutes and then he noticed me sitting there, my arms folded. "I expect you to know all this," he commented, looking right at me. So I started taking notes, lots of them, and halfway through the class my hand was hurting from writing. By the end of class, I had over ten pages of notes. His final words were to post our assignments on the class wiki and be ready to discuss them. I wondered how I would ever remember all the material from today, complete the assignment, and be ready for the next class. I wondered if I could do it.

The learning skills discussed in this chapter are ones that you will use every day. The first part of this chapter highlights the differences between high school and college. You will be encouraged to take action today to build a good foundation for success in the classroom. Next you will focus on five learning skills: time management, effective class notes, preparing for and taking tests, reading, and writing. Developing and practicing strong learning skills leads to success in the classroom as well as on the playing field. As you work through this chapter it is important to realize that this chapter is not about specific course content. It is about the learning skills that will help you be a successful student. If you need help today with a specific course, talk with the course instructor, teaching assistant, an academic tutor, or your coach. Do not wait.

Understanding How College Differs from High School

You have officially arrived. You are a collegiate student-athlete. You may be worried about the transition from high school sports to college-level sports; the competition is much tougher and the expectations are much higher. The same holds true for the academic side of the student-athlete equation. Things are just different.

In high school, you probably knew your teachers pretty well and were comfortable with the administrators, the school system, and the rules. You probably never had to give too much thought about what classes you were going to take and knew exactly who to turn to when you had a question or concern. Maybe your parents or guardians would nag you to do your homework, and maybe they filled out all the forms and paperwork that the school required. In college, the game changes a little, and it's up to you to navigate your own way.

To prepare you for the transition to college academics, here are a few changes that you can expect:

1. *Bigger class sizes:* You may have gone to a small high school or are accustomed to small class sizes where the teacher knows your name and you receive a lot of personal attention. At some colleges and universities, you may continue to have these small classes, but at many universities, classes can be quite large. You may find yourself in a big lecture hall with hundreds of other students. You may have classes where your professor doesn't know your name, and doesn't even take roll. Some students have a difficult time adjusting to larger class sizes. They may feel lost in a big class. They may be unmotivated by the lack of individual attention and start skipping classes because they think no one will notice or care. The reality is that if you're in a large class, it's even more important that you attend classes and monitor your own progress in the course. A helpful hint for finding success in a large class is to participate actively in class. Active participation requires that you attend class consistently, take thorough notes during lectures, attend any additional review sessions or study groups, and seek clarification for material you do not understand. If you have questions, visit the professor or teaching assistant during office hours. Make a point of getting to know classmates and consider joining a study group or working with a tutor if you need extra help.

2. *Diversity:* When you hear the word *diversity*, it is natural to think of skin color. However, diversity is much more. Diversity is in thought, size, education, gender, sexual orientation, economics/class status, geographic location, abilities/disabilities, and so on. Your classmates and teammates will be diverse. We go through life viewing other individuals based on what we know, have heard, have seen, or have been told. When we encounter people or a situation, we use our existing information about a group of people or a similar situation to determine how we will act (or react), what opinion we form, or what labels we will use. At times we do this without questioning if our information is factual, and often it isn't. College is a time to embrace differences and learn from people who have different views and beliefs.

3. *Choosing your own classes:* In high school, you may have had few options when it came to your class schedule. There were many required courses and your day was packed from morning through afternoon. In college, you have much more flexibility in terms of the courses that you take. You will have courses that are required for your major, but you will also have classes that you can take as electives. When choosing classes, there are two very important resources at your disposal—the college catalog and your academic adviser. Before choosing your classes, read the catalog and get a sense of what courses are needed to complete your degree. Also, determine in what order classes should be taken and when courses are offered. Meet with your academic adviser to map out a plan of action. This will help ensure that you fulfill all your academic requirements. Finally, when selecting courses, take into consideration who is teaching the class and when the class

is offered. For example, if you know that you have a hard time getting up in the morning and have a hard time focusing early in the day, it may not be a good idea to register for an 8:00 A.M. class.

4. *Managing your own time:* In high school your time was very structured. Perhaps a bus or a parent dropped you off at school the same time each morning and you had a set study hall. You may have had daily homework assignments to make sure that you were keeping up with your studies. In college, you have more freedom, and with that freedom greater responsibility. You are responsible for keeping up with your work, reading assignments, and getting to morning classes. As a student-athlete, you have even more to fit into your schedule. In addition to academics, you have practices, games, and team meetings. It becomes very important for you to learn how to budget your own time. It takes discipline to set aside time to go to the library or to read class assignments. It takes maturity to forgo a late-night outing with friends so that you can make sure that you get to bed early enough to make it to your early-morning class on time. You will not have a parent or guardian to bang on your door in the morning to make sure you are up in time for class; the responsibility is yours.

5. *Less-frequent tests:* As a high school student, you probably had weekly or even daily homework assignments. You probably also had several quizzes and tests for each class. In college there are fewer tests and assignments. Sounds like great news, right? On the surface, fewer tests seems like a blessing. But really, having fewer tests and assignments means that you have fewer checkpoints to see if you are on the right track. It also means a lot more individual reading and studying. As a college student, you will receive a course syllabus in the beginning of the semester. It will outline the material that will be covered in the course and it will also give the due dates for assignments and tests. Typically, college courses have only two or three tests or exams per semester. Courses may have a writing, research, lab, or participation component, but other than that, most of your final grade is derived from your score on two or three exams. With only a few tests, there are only a few chances for you to earn points toward your final grade. If you perform poorly on a test, it becomes difficult to dig yourself out of a hole. Here are some hints for adjusting to fewer tests and assignments:

   - Mark tests and assignments on your calendar. Don't let tests sneak up on you. As soon as you get your syllabus, identify tests and assignment due dates and budget your time accordingly.

   - Keep up with your reading. Don't put off your reading until the week before the exam—you will never get it all done in time.

   - Take good notes during class and review them periodically.

6. *More independent learning:* In high school, most teachers provide you with the materials you need to succeed. Teachers give you the information that you need to study for tests and

THINK ABOUT IT ✓

❑ What is one thing about college classes that is different from your high school classes? How will you adjust to this difference?

❑ Where does the information about people who are different from you come from? Family? Media? Personal experiences? Have you ever felt "different"?

❑ Describe a time when you performed really well in school; for example, you got an A on a final exam. What made you successful in that situation?

complete your assignments. Even in tough classes or advanced-level courses, your teacher probably laid out a framework for what was expected. Students can be successful without having to utilize many outside resources. In college, professors are less likely to provide you with all the facts and materials that you will need to succeed. Professors lay the framework for what you need to know, but they expect you to do additional reading, writing, and research on your own to get a fuller understanding of the subject matter. With more independent work and more critical thinking, analysis, and writing required, it is helpful for students to utilize campus resources such as the writing center, the reference desk, and the library. Take time when you first arrive on campus to become familiar with the campus library system. Learn how to use your library's online catalog system and how to conduct an Internet search.

Be a Proactive Learner

You are responsible for your academic success. To a large degree it will come down to your attitude and self-respect. There are a lot of opportunities and resources on a college campus. You need to believe that you can be and are a good student. Here are three actions you can take today to build a foundation to support your academic studies.

Be a Student First

As a student-athlete, you wear several hats. You are a student, an athlete, a son or daughter, a friend, a roommate, possibly a girlfriend or boyfriend, and maybe even an employee. It can be quite challenging to be all of these things at once, and it's particularly hard to be a dedicated student and an elite athlete at the same time. Often, student-athletes are forced to make hard decisions between sports and their commitment to their academics. Student-athletes are often pulled in two directions at once, and forced to choose one over the other. For example, you may have to choose between going to the training room with your teammate to get iced and stretched out before practice or sitting through a psychology lecture in an auditorium with a hundred other classmates. Which would you choose?

The bottom line is that you are a student first. Without being a student first and foremost, you would not even have the opportunity to be a collegiate athlete. Remember this when you have choices to make regarding your sports and school. Skipping a class today may not seem like a big deal, but things add up and if you do not give proper attention to your studies, you may find yourself doing poorly academically and may even find yourself ineligible to play. There will be times throughout the semester where sports may legitimately interfere with classes and school. There will be away games and travel that may take you away from your classes. It is unrealistic to think that on occasion, your involvement with sports will not interfere with or preempt your school work, but those instances should be the exception and not the rule. Remember that academic conduct is to be taken very seriously. Box 3.2 lists a few rules for academic conduct that must be upheld to maintain your status as a student-athlete.

Build Rapport with Professors

Professors will treat you as an adult and in turn they expect you to act as a mature, responsible individual. Professors are great people, but let's face it, they have busy schedules and are not in the business of holding students' hands. While they want you to succeed, they are not going to chase after you to make sure that you come to class or turn in your assignments. Rather, they expect you to seek them out if there is something you don't understand, if something is wrong,

STUDENT REFLECTION

Box 3.2. Academic Conduct

How is your academic conduct? Do you:

1. Attend classes regularly, complete all academic assignments, and adhere to the university's academic integrity guidelines?
2. Consult with academic advisers and attend tutoring sessions, as directed?
3. Maintain an academic load of at least twelve hours per semester and make satisfactory progress toward a degree, and accept responsibility for maintaining academic eligibility?
4. Complete at least six credits and attain the appropriate grade point average each semester?

or if you have a conflict with class. It is your responsibility to build a good working rapport with professors. To do so, you should be conscientious about your work, put forth your best effort, be honest, communicate openly, respect their time, and take their classes seriously. You will find that the respect you show will be reciprocated.

Playing a sport means that there will be the occasional conflict with class and assignments. It is important that you learn to handle such situations responsibly. Here are a few pointers for how to deal with a class conflict:

- *Find out what is expected from you by professors.* Each professor has his or her own set of rules regarding class structure, attendance, and grading. In the beginning of the semester, find out what the attendance policy is and when assignments and tests are due. See if there are any obvious conflicts between your athletic schedule and the course. If your professor has a very strict attendance policy and you already see that you will have to miss two classes due to games, you may wish to switch into another course that better fits your schedule or speak with your coach or adviser about other options.

- *Be up front with professors.* Make your professors aware of your schedule and involvement with athletics before there is a problem. At the start of the semester, e-mail your professors and let them know that you are a student-athlete but that academics are your first priority. If there are days that you will be out of town for away games or meets, let your professors know in advance. Apologize in advance for missing class and find out if there is anything that you can do to make up work.

- *Make up all work that you miss.* If you do have to miss a class, make up all the work that you missed as soon as possible. Ask for notes from a classmate or ask a friend to tape record the class lecture for you.

- *Be respectful of classroom policies.* If a professor has a rule about being on time for class or turning off cell phones in class, respect it. Do your best to uphold policies and don't ask for exceptions.

- *Don't make excuses!* You may think that the story about your dog eating your homework was pretty convincing, but professors weren't born yesterday. Don't lie about why you missed class or turned an assignment in late. You won't fool anyone. Professors will be much more understanding if you are honest and explain your situation. You are accountable for both your successes and your shortcomings, and showing ownership and responsibility is a sign of maturity that professors will respect.

There will be times that you have to make hard decisions regarding school and sports, and sometimes there has to be a compromise. It is important to speak to not only your professors but also your coaches about these conflicts.

Follow Academic Policies and Procedures

There is a laundry list of rules that you must follow in order to register for classes, be academically eligible to play sports, make academic progress, earn a degree, and graduate. Each school's policies and rules vary. This exercise will help you learn your school's academic rules. Use your school's Web site or your academic catalog to answer the questions below:

1. Who is your academic adviser?

2. How do you register for classes?

3. When is the add/drop period over?

4. How many classes/credit hours must you take each semester to play sports?

5. What GPA/QPA must you maintain to be eligible to play?

6. When and how can you declare a major?

7. Where can you find your degree requirements?

8. What happens if you withdraw from a class?

How to Manage Your Time

There are three main components of effective time management: planning your semester, making to-do lists, and utilizing a day planner. Using these three skills together will help you manage your time.

Plan Your Semester

Planning your semester requires that you take a step back and look at the big picture. To plan your semester:

- Purchase or download a monthly calendar so that you can see the entire semester at a glance.

THINK ABOUT IT

- ❑ Describe a time where sports conflicted with school. Did school or sports win out, and why?
- ❑ List three things you can do if you have to miss class due to an athletic event.

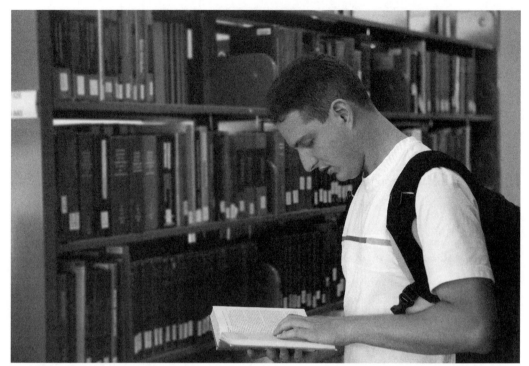

© Stephen Coburn/ShutterStock, Inc.

- Refer to your athletic schedule to identify dates that you have home games or competitions, travel, away games, tournaments, and any other special events that are related to your sport.

- Use your syllabi from all of your classes to identify when assignments are due or when you have tests and exams. Mark any special lectures or other important class dates on your calendar.

- Consult your school's academic calendar and add important academic dates and deadlines to your calendar. Include the add/drop deadline, spring break, course registration days, and other campus events on your calendar.

- Finally, mark any social commitments on your calendar. These include birthdays, parents' weekend, or events or activities that you plan in advance with friends or family.

- Look for conflicts in your schedule or things that overlap. For example, you may notice that you have a test in your art history class the same day that you are away for a soccer game. Once you have identified the conflict, you can plan accordingly. You should speak to your professor about this at the start of the semester and see if you can take the test early before you leave for your game, or discuss the situation with your coach and see if there is a way that you can be there for the test. The sooner you realize that you have a time conflict and address it, the more likely you will be to find a way to make your schedule work for you.

- Use your monthly calendar to help you schedule your day-to-day activities and plan for upcoming events and assignments.

Make To-Do Lists

Start each day by making a to-do list. Write down all the things that you wish to accomplish that day. Include in your list everything from reading chapters for class, to going to practice, to editing a paper, to meeting a friend for lunch, to watching the season premiere of your favorite television show.

Once you list all the things that you want to do that day, begin to prioritize your list. Identify things that you absolutely have to do, things that you would like to do if time permits, and things that you could postpone if you run out of time. Number the items on your list according to their importance. Star or highlight items that are absolutely necessary to complete so that you can focus your attention there.

As you go through your day, check off items that you complete; this will give you an amazing sense of accomplishment when you cross off one item after another. You will see exactly how productive you can be in a day. At the end of the day, assess how well you did. Create a game plan for how you are going to address any items that remain on your list. Maybe you will wake up early the next day and finish reading before class, maybe you will record your favorite television show and watch it over the weekend when you have more free time. Using a format similar to that in Box 3.3 will help you create an effective to-do list.

Use a Day Planner

The first step in managing your daily activity is purchasing a day planner. Your day planner should have a designated space for each day of the week, and that space should be divided into hour or half-hour increments. Fill out your day planner and include all scheduled activities for the day. Fit your classes, practice, meetings, appointments, and special events into the time slots. Include information like location so that you remember to give yourself enough time to travel from one activity to the next.

Once you have your daily schedule mapped out, you will be able to see gaps in your day where you can fit in items from your to-do list. For example, if you have class from 1:00 to 2:30

STUDENT REFLECTION

STUDENT REFLECTION

Box 3.3. To-Do List

Write all the things that you have to do today. Once you have identified all your to-do items, number them from 1–15 according to their level of priority or the order in which you will attempt to complete them.

Student Reflection: List up to 15 things you want   *Rank (1= most important to do)*
   to do today

_____

_____

_____

_____

_____

_____

_____

_____

_____

_____

_____

_____

_____

_____

_____

and don't have practice until 4:00, you may choose to fit in a quick trip to the bookstore, an item on your to-do list for the day. Mapping out your day and creating an hour-by-hour schedule will help you budget your time and avoid procrastination. You will have a visual representation of how you spend your time, which activities take up the majority of your time, and where you are likely to waste time.

Practice planning your day by completing the grid in Box 3.4. Be sure to account for all of your time.

Box 3.4. Seven-Day Plan: What Is Your Pattern?

Time	Monday	Tuesday	Wednesday	Thursday	Friday	Saturday	Sunday
5–6							
6–7							
7–8							
8–9							
9–10							
10–11							
11–12							
12–1							
1–2							
2–3							
3–4							
4–5							
5–6							
6–7							
7–8							
8–9							
9–10							
10–11							

THINK ABOUT IT ☑

❑ Post your semester plan on the wall of your room. Make it visible for you and others. Encourage your teammates to do the same with their schedules. At team study halls discuss your semester plan.

❑ Purchase 5 by 8 note cards and write your daily to-do list on the cards. Mark the items off as you complete them during the day. At the end of the day look at the card and see how you did. Use the card to plan the next day.

❑ Post the seven-day plan you created in this section on the wall of your room. Make it visible for you and others. Encourage your teammates to do the same. At team study halls discuss your seven-day plans. How are they the same and different?

How to Take Classroom Notes

Just going to class is not enough to be successful. To be a successful student, you must be an active learner in the classroom. This requires not only that you attend class, but also that you pay attention, ask questions, participate, and most important, take notes. Below are seven tips for being a successful learner in the classroom:

- *Be prepared for class:* Have a notebook or binder for each class. Label your notebooks or use different colors for different classes so that you don't accidentally grab the wrong one. Avoid writing notes on random pieces of paper. Scrap papers will inevitably get lost or your notes will fall out of sequence. Bring your notebook, binder, and any handouts or reading materials with you to every class. Also, have a pen or pencil with you, and keep a spare on hand. Bring a highlighter or an alternate color with you to class in case you want to emphasize something and make it stand out.

- *Be a good listener:* Taking notes begins with listening. To be a good listener, you should look at your instructor, sit up in your chair, and find a seat in the classroom where you can see the blackboard or screen and hear the instructor. Don't hide in the back of the classroom where you cannot see or hear.

- *Ask questions:* If you miss something that is said during class or you do not fully understand what was said, ask the professor to repeat the material. If you are uncomfortable asking professors to repeat themselves during a lecture, wait until after class and ask for clarification. If there is something missing in your notes or something that you are not sure that you wrote down correctly, you can also ask a classmate to compare notes with you to see if your notes are consistent with theirs. Make sure your notes are accurate and that you understand what was said during class. Professors tend to include much class material on tests and exams.

THINK ABOUT IT ✓

❑ Note taking is a study skill that requires practice. Note taking can be used during class lectures as well as when you read textbooks. The key to good note taking is being organized. Box 3.5 shows an example of how to organize notes. Use this format to go back and outline/take notes on this chapter.

• *Think through material:* Instead of simply writing down word for word what is said in class, it is helpful to think through what is said in class and relate it to what you already know. By thinking through material you can analyze and apply what you are learning, which will help you remember it and put it in a different context.

STUDENT REFLECTION

Box 3.5. Sample Outline for Formatting Notes

I. Class Information
    A. Class
    B. Instructor
    C. Date
    D. Chapters Covered
    E. Topic/Overall Theme

II. Main Idea
    A. Supporting Idea 1
        1. Examples:
        2. Vocabulary/Definitions:
        3. Keywords:
    B. Supporting Idea 2
        1. Examples:
        2. Vocabulary/Definitions:
        3. Keywords:
    C. Concepts/Theories:
    D. Applications:
        1. How does this information relate to previous knowledge?
        2. How does this information differ from what I already know?
        3. What makes this information significant?

- *Organize your notes:* Follow a consistent note-taking format. Use a numeric or alphabetical outline form, and underline vocabulary words that you define. Start new topics on a new page.

- *Stay alert and present:* Don't let your mind wander; keep your head up. Don't try to do other things like play on your laptop, text message, or read or finish assignments for another class. Don't try to read ahead; stay on the pace of your professor.

- *Be consistent:* Use the same method over and over and be consistent in all your classes. Don't skip a day. Even if you think you understand something, write it down. Even a brief description will jog your memory when it comes time to study.

How to Prepare for and Take Tests

An upcoming test can be a source of stress and anxiety for students. The key to being a good test taker lies in the preparation. How you prepare for a test has a direct impact on how well you perform. The first step in preparing for a test is knowing what to study. Make sure that you understand what your professor is expecting of you. Refer to your syllabus to see what chapters and topics will be included on the test. Make sure you know whether a test or exam is comprehensive and covers everything you have learned up until that point or whether it focuses on only a few chapters, the most recent work that you have done.

Once you have identified chapters and topics that will be included, identify key terms within those chapters and lessons. Define these terms and practice reciting and writing the definitions. You may wish to create a glossary of terms or write each key word on an index card or flash card. You can use flash cards to go over vocabulary and key terms throughout your day. For example, you can review definitions while waiting for the campus shuttle or on the bus ride to an away game.

In addition to identifying key words, also identify lists, diagrams, or charts that you covered in your reading or classes. Lists, diagrams, charts, and graphs may appear in an exam as a short answer or essay.

Match your study style to the exam format. If your professor says that the exam will be all essays, make sure you study large topics and main concepts. If the exam is multiple choice or true/false, focus on vocabulary, numbers, dates, or smaller details that the professor emphasized.

To study for a test or exam, do not wait until the night before. Give yourself extra time to go back through your class notes and readings, and determine what areas the professor emphasized, what areas are likely to be on the test, what areas you feel confident that you know, and what areas you really need to focus on. Giving yourself lead time before a test will allow you to organize your study materials, clarify anything you do not understand from your notes or readings, and make study review sheets or flash cards.

Finally, the day of your test, arrive early. If you are running late, you are less likely to be focused. Make sure you have a pen or pencil and any other needed supplies or materials with you. Before you begin, skim over the test. See the format and read all the directions. Decide how much time you can spend on each section. Be aware of how much time you have to complete the test. Do sections or questions that seem easy first. This will get you in the rhythm and will help you recall information that may help you answer more difficult questions. If you get stuck on a question, do not waste too much time. Move ahead and come back to it at the end.

Often a professor will tell the class what type of format will be used. For example, the test may be multiple choice, true/false, short answer, or essay. Depending on the format, you

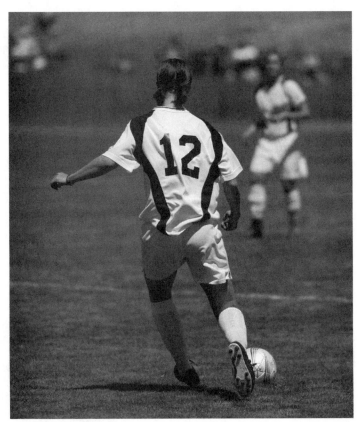

© Adam Tinney/ShutterStock, Inc.

should alter how you prepare and the strategy you take during the test. Sometimes, when students know in advance that a test is multiple choice, they study less because they think that the test will be easy because the answers will appear somewhere on the page. Multiple-choice tests aren't necessarily easier. Multiple choice actually allows professors to test on more specific and smaller pieces of information. In addition, the language of the questions may be confusing to you. When preparing for an objective multiple-choice test, try to identify topics, themes, and key words from your notes and text that may appear in a question. When taking a multiple-choice test, read questions carefully. Look for words like "always" or "never." Answers that say "always" or "never" are often incorrect. Watch out for whether they are asking for the right answer or the one answer that is not correct. Eliminate options that you know are incorrect to narrow your choices.

If answering a short-answer question or writing an essay, be direct, make your point, and then support your point. Don't waste time on filler sentences. It helps to outline your answer to an essay question before writing it. Doing so will ensure that your answer is organized and includes all your key points.

Answer all questions. Don't leave questions blank. Remember, there is always room for partial credit. Once you have answered all the questions, if time permits, go back and check your work. It is okay to use the entire time that a professor gives. Don't rush to finish just because other students may be finished and turning in their tests.

THINK ABOUT IT ✔

❑ Prepare a list of your upcoming tests for each of your classes. For each test complete the following information:

Material covered in test (chapters, assignments, readings, and class lectures)

Key words, diagrams, and charts.

Exam format (essay, short answers, multiple choice, true/false, fill in the blank). Is the exam written, oral, or computerized?

❑ Make a course test study schedule (same as a practice schedule for your sport). Determine when you will start with the fundamentals (i.e., key words, diagrams, charts), review your notes for each chapter, assignment, readings, and class lectures), and strategize how best to match your study plan with the test format (i.e., essay, short answer, multiple choice). Share your course test study schedule in your team study halls.

How to Read Textbooks

One of the main differences between high school and college academics is the level of independent learning that is required. Typically, college students are required to read independently prior to class. The amount of reading you will have to do in college is probably much greater than what you were used to in high school, and at first the amount may be overwhelming. Reading the texts, articles, journals, papers, and novels that are assigned for class is critical to being successful in the classroom. Professors often move through course material quickly and assume that everyone has read the corresponding text before coming to class. If you have not done your reading, it will be easy to fall behind. When you have a class a few times a week, it is hard to catch up. Therefore, it is extremely important that you stay on top of your reading. The last thing you want to do is cram an entire semester's worth of reading into a day or two just before an exam.

Reading for class is also important because professors will expect you to discuss what you read and learned during class. Many smaller classes will be driven by peer discussion. You will do yourself and your classmates a disservice if you do not read before class and come to class prepared to contribute to the discussion.

When you read, begin by previewing the chapter. Skim through the chapter, focusing on headings and bold words to get an idea of what you are going to be learning. Identify key topics or themes. Begin to draw on what you already know about the topic. For example, this chapter is about academics; before you started reading it, you should have recalled your own experiences as a student.

Read actively. Take notes or highlight important items. This will help you focus on critical points when you return to the text to study and review. Reread sections that are confusing. Note words that are defined and items that are listed. These items usually appear on tests and quizzes.

Reading the assigned literature is only the first step in studying. Studying is a process that takes place over the entire semester. Studying does not occur the day before a big exam—that is cramming! Studying requires consistent and repetitive learning of material. Studying requires that you read, rehearse, review, and retest yourself until you have memorized, understand, and can apply what you have learned.

Below are some helpful study tips:

Consider location: Have you ever heard the expression "location is everything"? Well, when it comes to studying, this statement holds true. When reading or studying, it is important that you find a quiet place without distractions. That place should have good lighting and plenty of table surface to spread out your materials. Become familiar with the library and visit it when you need to focus on your school work.

THINK ABOUT IT ✔

❑ Make space in your room for all of your class reading assignment materials (books, articles, papers, printouts of class notes, and assignments from the Internet). Typically, student-athletes like to keep them on a desk or a shelf above the desk.

❑ For each class, make a list of the readings. If your professors have electronic versions of the class readings on a schedule, print a copy for each class. Look at the readings to get an idea of what you are going to learn. Make and post a weekly schedule of your reading assignments on the wall of your room.

Stay alert: If you are dozing off while you're reading, you probably won't be very productive. After all, it's very hard to read with your eyes closed. Sit upright in a chair rather than lying on your bed or lounging in front of the television. Be an active reader by taking notes, outlining, or highlighting as you read. This will help you stay engaged with what you're reading.

Organize your study materials: Keep your notes, study sheets, and readings in a notebook, folder, or binder. When you sit down to study for an exam, have all your materials in front of you. Group reading and notes together by topic.

Jog your memory with creative memorization tricks: Memorization is an important part of studying. When you have lists of things to remember, it helps to use creative tricks such as making words or sayings out of the first letters of each item. For example, you may have an easier time remembering the five Great Lakes by remembering one word—HOMES—which stands for Lakes Huron, Ontario, Michigan, Erie, and Superior.

How to Write Papers

Writing papers in college can be an overwhelming task. Whether you have to write a two-page paper or a twenty-page paper, there are a few basic principles to follow. First and foremost, a paper is your opportunity to express a point and to support that point either with factual information that you have researched or with your own sound reasoning. Writing assignments are a great way to express what you have learned and utilize your creativity.

The first step in writing an effective paper is to create an outline. An outline will help you organize your thoughts and information and will serve as a road map for writing your paper.

Your outline should include the main point or topic, background information or an introduction, illustrative examples, analysis or synthesis, and a conclusion.

From your outline, you can begin to write your paper one paragraph at a time. Remember that paragraphs include an opening sentence, supporting sentences, and a concluding sentence. The opening sentence usually includes the topic of that paragraph. Make sure that you incorporate transition sentences from paragraph to paragraph so that your work flows and is easy for the reader to follow.

Content: Get your facts straight. Use the library and the Internet to research the topic that you are writing about and make sure that your facts are current.

Style: Follow the rules of the assignment. This includes adhering to page limits, font size and style, and margins. You must also be careful to adhere to academic policies regarding citing resources, quotes, or other people's work. If you use other people's writings, you must cite your sources to avoid plagiarism. If you have questions regarding how to properly cite someone else's work, visit your school's learning or writing center.

Accuracy: Finally, proofread your work. Go through what you have written and check for spelling and grammatical errors. Read your paper aloud so that you can hear how it sounds. Sometimes you can tell if a sentence is not structured properly or doesn't make sense if you stumble over it while reading it out loud.

If you are having difficulty writing a paper, visit the writing center or speak to the professor or teaching assistant for the class. Take advantage of the resources available to you at your school. After all, writing is a skill that must be developed over time and can always be improved with practice. Remember that writing is a process. You cannot write an entire paper in one sitting. You will need to make several drafts and revisions.

There are six key steps to writing an effective paper:

1. Brainstorm

2. Outline

3. Write a first draft

4. Make revisions

5. Edit

6. Do a final proof read

THINK ABOUT IT ✔

❏ Write a three paragraph essay (each paragraph with four to six sentences) on the pro and cons of being a college student-athlete. Follow the guide below to go through the first three steps of the writing process (Brainstorm, Outline, and Write First Draft)

A. Brainstorm: Write down what comes to minds when you think about the positive things about being a student-athlete.

_____

_____

_____

_____

_____

List all of the negative things or things that you dislike about being a student-athlete.

_____

_____

_____

_____

_____

B. Outline: Organize your thoughts into an outline.

   I.   Paragraph 1: Introduce Topic

_____

_____

   II. Make First Point

_____

_____

      i.   Support First Point

_____

_____

ii.   Support

_____

_____

iii. Support

_____

_____

III. Paragraph 2: Transition

_____

_____

   i.   Second Point:

_____

_____

      1.   Support Second Point:

_____

_____

      2.   Support:

_____

_____

      3.   Support:

_____

_____

IV. Paragraph 3: Conclusion

_____

_____

_____

_____

C. Write First Draft: On a separate piece of paper write a short essay, using your outline as a guide.

PLUGGED IN TO SPORTS

Student-Athletes and Technology

Technology is changing how we learn. College and university professors use a variety of Internet-based education support systems and methods. Depending on your school the name will vary (e.g., Blackboard Academic Suite, Oncourse CL, Stellar CourseWork, CT Tools, Elyon). Professors also use PowerPoint presentations, blogs, video clips, recordings, films, and laptops in the classroom. Some students bring their laptops to class, take notes, and at times might be able to follow along with the lecture on the Internet. Most college students register for classes online, correspond with professors and classmates through e-mail, and view their grades and academic progress on a computer. Technology can definitely enhance academics and the learning experience, but what happens when technology invades the classroom? Cell phones vibrate during class, students are playing computer games or instant messaging during class, iPods are playing in the back of a lecture hall. The use of technologies like these has gotten so distracting that many professors have actually added policies regarding phones and games during class to the syllabi.

One example of responsible use of electronics in the classroom is using the recording capabilities of cell phones, iPods, and MP3 players to distribute audio materials, such as famous speeches; recording interviews and field notes; and facilitating oral exercises, such as repetition of Spanish vocabulary words. Students can also use such devices to view pictures and movies, listen to Podcasts, and use other educational supplements prior to lecture, allowing class time to be entirely devoted to discussion. In fact, by creating a Podcast, students can have automatic access to course materials on their iPods or download them to their portable MP3 player.

Finally, be wary of technology overload and unlimited access to course materials; they could make class attendance seem unnecessary and obsolete. There is now a danger through technology that students may become distance learners even while on campus. And missing class is the first step toward not doing well in a class.

Chapter Summary

A major difference between high school and college or between a two-year college and four-year institution is how classes are taught and their degree of difficulty. Even if you have taken advanced placement classes in high school, you may find college-level courses challenging because they require you, not your instructor, to be responsible for what is learned. You are responsible for attending classes, for turning in your assignments on time, and for adequately preparing yourself for exams. The decision of whether you do these things is completely your own.

As a student-athlete you already possess many skills and strengths that can help you to be successful in your classes. Five learning skills were discussed in this chapter: time management, taking effective class notes, preparing for and taking tests, reading, and writing. You may need to work more on developing a particular learning skill. You can talk with a course instructor, coach, academic support counselor, family member, or friend to develop and strengthen your learning skills further.

Your Thoughts

1. Recall a time when it was difficult for you to manage sports and academics. Given what you learned in this chapter, identify ways that you could better handle that situation today.

2. What would you say to a teammate who made a derogatory joke or statement, or used words about another person, that made you uncomfortable enough that you didn't want to be around your teammate?

3. Student-athletes tend to be competitive, focused, disciplined, and determined. How can these attributes help you to be a better student? What are some other skills or attributes that you have as a student-athlete that you can apply to the classroom?

4. What advice can you give to a friend or teammate who is having difficulty making a realistic schedule?

5. Identify some pitfalls or distractions that prevent you from staying on task and adhering to your schedule. What can you do to overcome them?

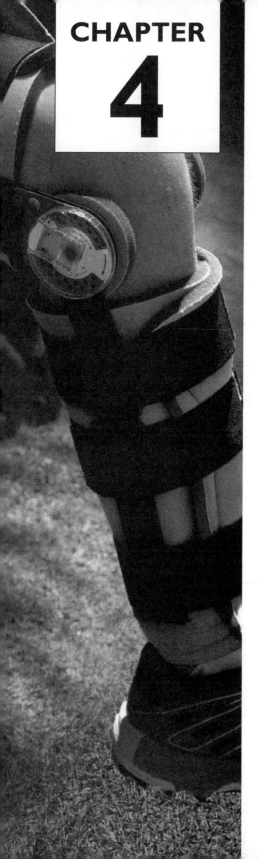

CHAPTER 4

Challenge #2: Pain and Injury

Learning Objectives

After completing this chapter, you will be able to:

- *Understand the differences between chronic and acute pain*

- *Discuss pain thresholds and the decisions that student-athletes face regarding whether or not to play through pain*

- *Identify different types of pain medications and understand the risks associated with them*

- *Understand how to prevent injury and seek treatment for injuries by working with coaches, trainers, and medical professionals*

- *Understand the emotional and mental effects of injury and how to cope with performance setbacks*

Student-Athletes Say:

- I dislocated both of my shoulders and needed surgery. It was emotionally painful to know I would not be able to play until the next season.

- Throughout my gymnastics career, I have had multiple stress fractures in my shins and back. I am constantly battling an injury.

- In my freshman year, I made it to the conference championship for track. When running in the semifinals for the 200, I felt my hip pop out of its socket. Even though I could hardly walk, I finished the race.

- Getting up at 5:45 A.M. even once a week to lift is painful.

- I sprained my ankle playing tennis and my doctor prescribed a high dose of ibuprofen. I used it every day before practice. When I finally stopped taking it, I felt awful. My entire body hurt. I needed the ibuprofen to compete.

- I tore my ACL and had to have knee surgery. I feel invisible, as if I am no longer part of the team. I hate that there is someone else out there playing my position. The worst part is worrying if I'll ever recover enough to play again.

If you play sports, you are going to have aches, pains, or injuries. There is no way around it for college student-athletes. Depending on the circumstances, the experience of pain can produce vastly different physical and psychological perceptions and responses. After a hard practice you may hurt: maybe every bone and muscle in your body aches, but overall you feel good. You worked hard and you are excited about the upcoming competition. It is going to be fun. This pain (sometimes called performance pain) is perceived as acute, short in duration, produced voluntarily, under your control, and you can reduce it by pushing less, reducing your training, speed, and activity. The feelings produced are positive—satisfaction, improved performance, and an enhanced sense of well-being. Performance pain is perceived as positive and reinforces your efforts and inspires a higher level of training and competition.

Pain from an injury is different. Injury pain is commonly experienced as chronic, long lasting, uncontrollable, and a signal of danger to physical well-being, and it motivates athletes to protect injured areas. Often a student-athlete's response to injury pain is a loss of confidence and motivation, increased anxiety and/or depression, and feelings of fear and dread. Injury pain is seen as negative and discouraging. Describing the pain from an injury, athletes tend to talk about acute and chronic pain. Acute pain is due to trauma and is intense but short in duration.

It is a warning to the body of damage and the need for immediate attention. Chronic pain is more complex. It is long lasting and persists beyond the injury. Chronic pain is often accompanied by physical, psychological, and social consequences.

Another way to think about pain is whether it is simply a benign artifact of the demands you are placing on an injured area or an important signal of further harm. Benign pain is typically characterized as dull, generalized, not lasting long after exertion, and not attended by swelling, localized tenderness, or lasting soreness. Harmful pain, in contrast, is considered to be sharp, localized to an injured area, experienced during and persisting after exertion, and usually associated with swelling, localized tenderness, and prolonged soreness.

This chapter focuses on the information and skills you need to meet the pain and injury challenge. As a student-athlete you may live with pain. To get started, complete the Student-Athlete Challenge # 2: Pain and Injury Self-Assessment in Box 4.1. Think about your lifetime experience with pain and injuries. In high school and maybe even earlier in your life, did you have a serious injury that prevented you from playing sports? How do you react when teammates are injured and in pain?

If you are not in pain or injured, then one of your teammates is. Often pain and injury is so accepted and expected that you do not even give it a second thought. It is not a reason not to practice or to compete. Modern medicine, physical therapy, and appliances (e.g., knee brackets, tape) make it possible to play through pain and injury. However, you must always ask yourself, "Is playing with pain and injury the best for me?" It is your choice.

My sophomore year started with a lot of back pain and three cortisone injections. I'm a 125-pound female, and the doctor gave me a dose of pain medication typically prescribed for a 200-pound male because my pain just wouldn't go away. After the shots, I returned to practice because the medication did the trick. It was great. I had no pain during most of the season. Over time my back pain started to come back and I had to go for another cortisone shot. After that shot, I couldn't feel my leg; it was completely numb. I freaked out and called my parents. They said I should quit competing because I was literally paralyzing myself. I told them no, gymnastics is my life and has been since I was two years old. After a couple of hours, I started to feel better because the pain medication was kicking in, but later in the week I noticed that I couldn't run without limping. I was not able to compete in the floor, vault, and beam events because I could not push off my foot. Over the year, I got the feeling and strength back in my leg with a lot of rehab. During my junior year, I was able to compete only in the bars event. I still had pain, but it was bearable. Now, in my senior year, I can't run or do any exercise that causes pressure or pounding. I'm usually limited to the elliptical or stepper to stay in shape. When we do plyometric work-outs as a team, my body hurts for the next two days. I have two herniated discs, and a spot in my back where there is no cartilage left and there is just bone rubbing on bone. As a freshman, I felt so much pride being a star gymnast. I felt my pride being torn apart when I was no longer able to compete in all four events. I'm at the point now where I don't even like gymnastics anymore because I can't do it without pain. That makes me miserable. This sport is my life and it paid for my school.

Box 4.1. Student-Athlete Challenge #2: *Pain and Injury Self-Assessment*

Directions: Evaluate each statement on a scale of 1 to 5, from 1 being "never" to 5 being "almost always." For each statement evaluate if your behavior adds value (+), is neutral (0), or decreases value (−) of your student-athlete success in regards to your classes and sport.

Statement	Never				Almost Always	Value Added		
	1	2	3	4	5	+	0	−
1. I take medication such as acetaminophen or ibuprofen to push through physical pain.	❏	❏	❏	❏	❏	❏	❏	❏
2. I don't mention the pain that I experience during practice and competition.	❏	❏	❏	❏	❏	❏	❏	❏
3. I feel like I am always injured and never able to compete at my highest level.	❏	❏	❏	❏	❏	❏	❏	❏
4. Injuries affect me not only physically but socially and emotionally as well.	❏	❏	❏	❏	❏	❏	❏	❏
5. An injury or having pain has made me feel socially withdrawn or depressed.	❏	❏	❏	❏	❏	❏	❏	❏
6. I know my body's limits and I don't push through pain that could cause a serious injury.	❏	❏	❏	❏	❏	❏	❏	❏
7. I go to the trainer's room before practice.	❏	❏	❏	❏	❏	❏	❏	❏
8. Even when I am injured, I try to stay involved with the team and still attend practices.	❏	❏	❏	❏	❏	❏	❏	❏
9. Coaches and trainers are understanding and supportive of my situation when I am injured.	❏	❏	❏	❏	❏	❏	❏	❏
10. I take the necessary steps to lower my risk of injury (warmup, stretch, good diet, cooldown)	❏	❏	❏	❏	❏	❏	❏	❏
11. I ice my body after practice and competitions.	❏	❏	❏	❏	❏	❏	❏	❏
12. I have been ridiculed or looked down upon for complaining about an injury.	❏	❏	❏	❏	❏	❏	❏	❏

Typically, pain is perceived as an unpleasant experience meant to be avoided. However, pain (and injury) is part of your world as a student-athlete. This chapter focuses on how pain is assessed and how different types of pain feel and affect you physically and psychologically. Understanding pain enables you to use the information to mange your pain and collaborate with coaches, athletic trainers, and other health professionals in addressing your concerns. Finally, understanding pain enhances your perceptions of control, which may have substantial physical and psychological benefits.

Understanding Your Body's Limitations

The Nature of Pain

Pain is best known and characterized as a subjective phenomenon. The function of pain is to indicate that something in the body is wrong. The nature of pain encompasses a more global and conceptual view. Pain is a universal human experience. Like a defense mechanism, pain is valuable to the body's response to invasion from germs, diseases, injury, and illnesses because it is one of the body's most important protective devices and a strong motivator for action. The feeling of pain is a natural response to injury or bodily harm, and it is the most common reason people request medical care. Pain is defined as an unpleasant sensory, physical, and emotional experience that is associated with actual or potential damage to the body. The human body is fragile, and most people do not know how to emotionally ignore pain. Thus, it is important to discuss both the physical and psychosocial responses to it.

Pain is more than just a physical sensation caused by a specific stimulus. Pain also has emotional and cognitive components. The physical component of pain includes bumps, breaks, and bruises that occur when stress and emotional demands impact the body. For example, if you get hit in the face by a ball, you will experience physical pain that will manifest itself through a bruise, puffiness, and redness. Emotional and cognitive components of pain are a little more abstract, and include anxiety, embarrassment, and worry or loss of the satisfaction or pleasure. For instance, many people participating on a team might feel anxiety and embarrassment if they miss the game-winning shot.

Additionally, scientifically there are two components of pain: emotional and physical. Physical pain can be broken down into two types. The first is direct pain, which is caused by the stimulation of nerve endings in an affected area. Direct pain is often associated with physical pain, where injury occurs to a specific area of the body. The second type is referred pain, where pain emerges in one place while the source or cause of the pain is elsewhere. For example, someone who is experiencing a heart attack may not only feel pain in their chest, but also have pain in their arm or tension in their jaw.

The most frequent pain that many student-athletes encounter numerous times and at many different levels during their athletic career is direct pain and injury to their bodies. Student-athletes push their bodies and minds to the limit each day to reach their performance goals, often while experiencing pain. Most student-athletes keep rigorous athletic and academic schedules, thus they do not take enough time to rest or recuperate. The emotional pain and disappointment of not being able to perform at their best is often as painful to them as their physical injuries. For example, during the 1996 Olympics, a young gymnast named Kerri Strug attempted her final vault even though she had hurt her ankle and could barely walk. Her determination and emotional spirit drove her to overcome her physical pain and finish the competition. For her, the idea giving up on her Olympic dreams was just as painful as tearing tendons in her leg.

Pain Tolerance, Threshold, and Assessment

Physiologically, the human body is designed to handle certain levels of pain. Therefore, people are capable of blocking out a degree of pain or discomfort without it influencing their performance. When engrossed in physical activity, some people are able to ignore pain; however, most can only ignore it for a short time. During intervals of high stress or pain, the brain secretes chemicals called opioids that act as powerful numbing agents. High levels of opioids give people a heightened tolerance for pain. This phenomenon was observed by battlefield surgeons who found that severely wounded soldiers needed lower doses of narcotics to handle their pain compared with civilians with far less serious injuries. Similarly, student-athletes can handle pain better than the average person during intense competitions because they are expected to tolerate a higher level of pain.

The body responds to different types of stress and pain in different ways. Because acute pain is experienced for a short time, unlike long-term or chronic pain, the body is more likely to adapt to it. For example, when you land on your ankle the wrong way, the body first reacts to this pain quickly, then braces you from the initial feeling of pain, and finally warns you that something is wrong. If you continue to play and reinjure your ankle after landing on it wrong, you may now sprain it, and the pain can become chronic. Chronic pain can last for weeks, months, or even years; however, your response to acute pain will determine if it becomes chronic. Thus, you should use the RICE (rest, ice, compress, and elevate) technique when you have an injury instead of playing through the pain.

Personal attitudes, beliefs, and societal influences also impact how a person perceives pain and how he or she reacts to injury. A person who becomes injured needs to evaluate his or her pain threshold and decide whether to push through the pain or to seek treatment. This is a very difficult decision for people who are motivated to work hard and do not want to alter their daily regimen. Gender differences and cultural messages have a significant impact on pain thresholds. For instance, males are typically told and encouraged to push their bodies through pain; any sign of weakness is considered feminine. Athletes in particular, both male and female, are also notorious for being conditioned to play through the pain. Frequently, they may be afraid of disappointing their teammates and being perceived as weak. As a result, many athletes take risks with their bodies, trying to play longer and harder despite any physical pain or setbacks they may be experiencing. Eventually, the decision to continue playing even when pain persists can have detrimental short- and long-term impacts on the body such as discontinued participation in athletic performances or even difficulty with daily activities. As a result, the athlete is eventually the only one who has to deal with the negative results of playing through pain.

As a student-athlete, it is critically important to be aware of your body's limitations because ignoring physical pain for too long can result in serious injury. In reality, however, it is also imperative that student-athletes strive to perform at their best and achieve physical goals. Thus, athletes need to acknowledge the signs and symptoms of short intervals of pain and they need to be careful not to ignore prolonged pain and injury. For example, David was a star hockey player at a local university. During playoffs, David got hit by a teammate and hurt his finger during practice. At the end of practice, David was in excruciating pain. One of his teammates told him to see the athletic trainer, but David knew that the trainer would probably tell him not to play and he would miss the first playoff game. Instead, David took ibuprofen and got back on the ice the next day. During the first play of the game, David was hit while fighting for the puck. Immediately, he fell to the ice. When the athletic trainer removed his glove, it was obvious that his finger was broken in several places. The health care provider had to splint David's hand, and as a result, he missed the rest of the postseason. If David had acknowledged his initial pain and sought treatment, he may have prevented the break and had a less severe injury.

THINK ABOUT IT

- ❑ As a student-athlete do you feel pressure from coaches, family, teammates, or fans to play through pain and injury?

- ❑ Do you have a plan for managing the pain you experience regularly from the rigors of training? How does this plan fit into your schedule?

- ❑ Describe a situation where you or a teammate ignored physical limitations and pushed your body beyond the limits. What was the result of not listening to the pain you or your teammate felt?

Working with Your Health Care Providers and Team Trainers

Health care providers and team trainers have different perspectives on pain, different knowledge bases or skills to diagnose chronic pain conditions, and differing capabilities or differing "tools" in their own personal toolbox, so people with chronic pain must understand that different caregivers may give them different diagnoses and different treatment plans. Student-athletes should also know that not all health care providers know all of the possible "tools of the trade" to treat student-athletes in pain. Some providers and trainers only practice noninvasive pain management and others offer only invasive therapies. Some offer both noninvasive and invasive therapies in their practice.

Pain is a complex condition that can affect you in several ways. Besides making your body hurt, pain can "hurt" your overall health and emotional well-being. It can make you feel isolated, anxious, or depressed. Pain can also stop you from doing things you enjoy, affect your ability to work, and keep you from sleeping well or eating right. Pain can even interfere with your relationships with family and friends.

It's important to understand that pain is a medical condition that can—and should—be treated. In this way, pain is similar to other medical problems, like infections, high blood pressure, or diabetes. You should expect to be treated for pain much as you would expect treatment for these other types of medical conditions.

But, the health care provider and trainers can't see or detect your pain. This is why it's up to you to tell them you're in pain and to describe your pain as clearly and specifically as possible. And, ultimately, it's up to you to ask for help.

The more you tell your health care provider about your pain and how it affects your life, the more he or she will be able to help you. And the more you learn about pain management, the more control you will have over your pain.

Talking about your pain requires you to talk about the pain as well as feel comfortable that you and your health care provider are doing all that can be done to address your needs. Keep in mind that pain management is a partnership among you, your health care provider, and other professionals who may be involved. The American Pain Association (www.pain foundation.org) recommends that you be assertive in your treatment. This includes preparing to talk about your pain prior to treatment and therapy as well as questions to ask during treatment and therapy. It's up to you to take control of your pain management and be an active partner.

Preparing to Talk About Your Pain

Since your health care provider can't see or detect your pain, it's your responsibility to make sure he or she has a clear understanding of how you feel. You need be ready to tell the physician, athletic trainer, physical therapist, or other health care provider about your pain in as much detail as possible.

- *Where is your pain?* Describe all painful areas.

- *How bad is your pain?* Give the health care provider specific information about the pain you feel. Use descriptive words, like *throb, ache, burn,* or *tingle.* Is your pain mild, moderate, or severe? Are you constantly in pain, or does it come and go? Does it vary in intensity? What, if anything, triggers your pain (for example, moving a particular way, doing certain tasks, changes in weather, stressful situations)? Is your pain bearable, or is it excruciating?

- *What do you think causes your pain?* In many situations, you will know the exact source of the pain (i.e., you'll know if it is a practice or a competition-specific injury). With some pain the cause will be more obtuse, appearing, for example, with prolonged exertion or a particular movement.

- *How long have you been in pain?* Think back over the course of your athletic career and be ready to talk about prior injuries and pain to provide a context and history.

- *How do you relieve your pain?* Describe ways you've learned to make your pain feel better, such as using heat, stretching, or taking nonprescription drugs like aspirin, acetaminophen, or ibuprofen.

- *What pain medications have you taken in the past?* Describe any past experiences with pain medications and how well they worked. Also mention any side effects you experienced, particularly stomach upset, heartburn, or gastrointestinal distress. Some prescription pain medications can cause constipation, nausea, dizziness, headache, drowsiness, and vomiting. Later in this chapter these medications are discussed in detail.

- *Besides pain, what other medical conditions do you have?* Make sure the health care provider is aware of all conditions you have, such as ulcers, high blood pressure, diabetes, kidney problems, or depression. Also make sure the health care provider is aware of all medications you take, including those that you buy without a prescription. Some pain medications are dangerous if they are taken with other types of drugs. Others can contribute to conditions like stomach distress or kidney problems.

- *Do you have any allergies?* Some pain medications can cause allergic reactions. Make sure your health care provider knows about any allergies or drug reactions you've experienced.

- *Do you have any fears or concerns about pain medications?* Many student-athletes are reluctant to take pain medications because of concerns about side effects. Others are worried they'll become "hooked" or addicted. Discuss your concerns with your health care provider.

- *Has your pain forced you to make changes in your lifestyle?* Let your health care provider know how your pain has affected your emotions and behavior. Has it affected your ability to concentrate, attend class, attend practice, and compete? Has it made you feel angry or sad? Has it affected your personal relationships?

Questions to Ask Your Health Care Providers and Team Trainers

The more you understand about the pain therapy your health care provider recommends, the more you will benefit from the treatment. Don't hesitate to ask any questions you may have. Remember, your health care provider wants to help. Here are some questions you should ask:

- *How well do you (trainer, therapist, physician) understand the pain I feel?* Discuss the answers to the above questions. The more your health care provider understands about your pain, the better he or she will be able to treat you.

- *Do I need to see a specialist?* Certain types of pain require the attention of a medical specialist, such as a neurologist, physiatrist, or orthopedic surgeon. There are also health care providers who specialize in treating pain, and pain clinics that offer comprehensive pain management programs. Finding the right health care provider and the right pain management program is critical to the success of your treatment.

- *Will pain medicine help me?* Several types of pain medications are available to relieve pain, including NSAIDs (nonsteroidal anti-inflammatory drugs), tramadol, and other centrally acting analgesics. Not all pain medications work effectively in all student-athletes. Tell your health care provider immediately if you're not getting adequate relief from prescribed medication. Also tell your health care provider if the side effects of your therapy are bothersome—or unacceptable. Work with your health care provider to find the therapy that's best for you. This may mean adjusting the dose, or switching to a different type of pain medicine. Keep in mind that medication is only one aspect of effective pain management. Ask your health care provider if non-drug treatments such as physical therapy, exercise, or relaxation techniques would be helpful in your case.

- *Do pain medications cause side effects?* Most pain medications cause side effects, some more serious than others. The commonly prescribed NSAID pain relievers irritate the lining in the stomach and intestines, which can cause ulcers or gastrointestinal bleeding. The other types of commonly prescribed pain drugs have different kinds of side effects, including constipation, drowsiness, nausea, vomiting, or dizziness. Side effects sometimes occur when you begin therapy and go away after your body gets used to the medication. Certain types of pain medicine can also cause physical dependence.

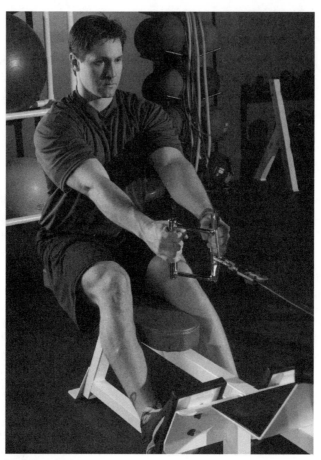

© Yuri Arcurs/ShutterStock, Inc.

- *Do pain medications cause seizures?* Although uncommon, there is a risk of seizure associated with some centrally acting analgesics. It is important to tell your health care professional if you have previously had a seizure and if you are taking opioid analgesics or medications commonly used to treat depression (e.g., amitriptyline, fluoxetine). Also, taking pain medications above the recommended dosage increases the risk of seizures.

- *Should I take other medication to manage the side effects of my pain therapy?* While taking medications to relieve the side effects of pain therapy may offer temporary relief, it could also disguise a serious medical problem. Many student-athletes, for example, take antacids or acid blockers to ease stomach distress caused by NSAIDs. But masking gastrointestinal symptoms can lead to critical delays in detection and treatment of emergency complications, such as ulcers.

- *Will I become addicted to pain medication?* Information indicates that getting "hooked on" or addicted to pain medication is rare. It's true that certain pain medications can cause physical dependence, which means the student-athlete may feel flulike or have other types of "withdrawal symptoms" when medication is stopped. In most cases, these symptoms can be avoided through gradual withdrawal based on increasingly smaller doses. It's important to understand that physical dependence does not mean abuse or addiction. Certain pain medications can be used inappropriately (abused) to get high or for effects other than pain relief. Addiction is a psychological problem that compels student-athletes to abuse pain drugs. Don't let any misunderstandings of the difference between physical dependence, abuse, and addiction prevent you from getting the most effective relief for your pain.

- *Can I take nonprescription pain relievers in addition to prescription pain drugs?* Sometimes, student-athletes have intensified bouts of pain that are not controlled by otherwise effective pain therapy. If this happens, you may be tempted to take nonprescription drugs for added relief. But first ask your health care provider or pharmacist if it's safe. Combinations of certain pain relievers could cause serious problems.

- *Besides taking medicine, what else can I do to manage my pain?* Pain medication is only one aspect of effective pain management. Your health care provider might suggest several types of non-drug treatments in addition to drug therapy. Non-drug treatments include physical therapy, acupuncture, exercise, breathing and relaxation techniques, biofeedback, massage, hot or cold packs, or nerve stimulation through a technique called transcutaneous electrical nerve stimulation (TENS). Your health care provider might also suggest changes in your diet. Ask your health care provider to discuss the types of non-drug pain management approaches that might help you.

Pain can make you feel sad, angry, vulnerable, lonely—or a host of other negative emotions. Many student-athletes have learned to cope with these emotions through professional counseling or student-athlete support groups. Ask your health care provider for help in finding these services.

Student-athletes respond to pain in different ways. Some student-athletes even believe that acknowledging pain is a character weakness. Keep in mind that pain is a medical condition. You should expect to be treated for pain just like you expect treatment for other medical problems. But remember, it's your responsibility to ask your health care provider to help you control your pain. Don't hesitate to ask your health care provider for help. And don't hesitate to ask your health care provider questions about the pain management approach he or she recommends.

THINK ABOUT IT

- ❑ What can you do to ensure that you get all your questions regarding your injury and treatment answered?
- ❑ What services are available for you on campus if you need medical treatment or special accommodations for an injury?

Pain Medication Options

Relieving the physical sensation of pain with medication is an important step in managing pain. Several types of pain medications are available that relieve both acute and chronic pain. But medications work differently for different people. Some may not give you the pain relief you need. Some may treat your underlying condition, not your pain. Others have serious side effects you should know about before you agree to take them. Most forms of student-athlete sports-related pain respond to non-opioid drug treatments such as aspirin, acetaminophen, ibuprofen, naproxen, and other NSAIDs. However, prescription pain medication sometimes will be used to treat pain.

It's also important to understand that medication is only one type of medical treatment for pain and only one aspect of successful pain management. In fact, studies increasingly show that pain management is most effective when it is based on a multidisciplinary approach that addresses the emotional and behavioral consequences of pain as well as the physical discomfort.

NSAIDs and Over-the-Counter Analgesics

Discovered in 1897 by Felix Hoffman at the Bayer Company in Germany, the first pain medication utilized in the Western world was aspirin. Currently, there are more pain medications to choose from than aspirin. In fact, most pain medications are easily accessible over the counter because they are nonprescription medications—part of a billion-dollar drug industry in America.

The four main classifications of over-the-counter drugs (OTCs) are aspirin, acetaminophen, ibuprofen, and naproxen. Of these, aspirin, ibuprofen and naproxen are referred to as NSAIDs (nonsteroidal anti-inflammatory drugs). These drugs reduce the swelling and inflammation often associated with injury or illness. Unlike cortisone-based steroids often prescribed to relieve inflammation, NSAIDs are nonsteroidal. Alternatively, acetaminophen is classified not as an NSAID but rather as an analgesic, because it does not reduce inflammation. The three applications of NSAIDs are relieving mild to moderate pain, such as headaches; reducing inflammation and tenderness in joints; and lowering elevated body temperature when the body fights infection, such as a fever. Box 4.2 provides some questions to review your knowledge of NSAIDs and OTC analgesics.

The most common NSAID, aspirin, can reduce fever and relieve minor aches and pains. While aspirin is helpful, there are side effects associated with it that may be problematic, such as developing gastric bleeding in the stomach if taken in large amounts. Aspirin also increases the time it takes for blood to clot. This reduction in clotting, also known as thinning of the blood, can be beneficial for student-athletes who are susceptible to small clots, which block coronary arteries; however, it can also be dangerous because it increases the risk of hemorrhaging or excessive bleeding if someone is cut.

STUDENT REFLECTION

Box 4.2. How Much Do You Know About Pain Medication?

Check your understanding of NSAIDs and OTC analgesic drugs by associating the following characteristics with (a) aspirin, (b) acetaminophen, (c) ibuprofen, or (d) naproxen. Some characteristics may be applicable to more than one category of OTC analgesic drug.

1. A common brand name of this drug is Tylenol
2. Reduction of inflammation is one of the medical applications of this drug
3. Gastric distress is most severe with this drug
4. Combination of this drug with alcohol can lead to serious liver damage
5. This drug has an anti-clotting effect
6. Blocking the production of prostaglandins is a physiological effect of this drug
7. This drug is the oldest known of the four types of analgesic drugs

Answers: 1-b; 2-a, c, & d; 3-a; 4-b; 5-a, c, & d; 6-a & c; 7-a

Similarly, ibuprofen is another NSAID that has been approved by the Food and Drug Administration (FDA) to be sold over the counter. Advil, Motrin, and Nuprin are among the most common brand names of ibuprofen. Along with aspirin, ibuprofen can reduce pain, inflammation, and elevated temperatures. It has also been successful in suppressing menstrual cramp pain. Unlike aspirin, ibuprofen appears to cause less gastric irritation; however, prolonged usage can create the potential for kidney damage or failure.

Naproxen, also known by the brand name Aleve, is the newest OTC analgesic drug on the market. Naproxen has the same effect as aspirin and ibuprofen; however, active ingredients last for eight to twelve hours, a substantially longer time period than the other types of OTC analgesics. The chief complaint with naproxen is gastrointestinal irritation. Chronic use may cause gastric bleeding, ulceration, or perforation of the stomach wall.

Lastly, one of the most popular OTC analgesics is acetaminophen, which is sold under the brand names Tylenol, Datril, and Anacin-3. Even though acetaminophen is not an anti-inflammatory drug, it is a popular alternative to aspirin and ibuprofen. Unlike the other OTCs, acetaminophen does not produce gastric distress or interfere with the clotting process; however, it is not entirely free of adverse side effects. It is known to have a relatively high potential for causing liver damage. This occurs with large doses, chronic use, or combined use with alcohol and other drugs. In fact, taking acetaminophen after a weekend drinking binge can prove fatal. The amount of toxic reaction varies from person to person, and thus it is not possible to give guidelines for safe alcohol ingestion with acetaminophen use.

Student-athletes can become addicted to pain medications if they use them for long periods of time. For instance, David, the ice hockey player mentioned earlier, was told by his health care provider to take aspirin to alleviate the pain he was feeling from his injury. Long after David's broken finger healed, he still experienced discomfort and continued to take aspirin daily. After a few months, David began to experience stomach pain. He went back to his health care provider and found out that the aspirin, which he was taking up to three times a day, was eating away at his stomach lining and causing internal bleeding. Examples like this show us that overuse or dependency on pain medications may lead to serious health consequences.

Prescription Pain Medicine

Prescription pain medication is derived from opiates. Examples of opioid pain medications are oxycodone, morphine, and codeine. And while these prescription pain medications are very effective for pain management, the risk of dependency or addiction is a concern for both student-athletes and prescribing physicians.

If you believe you are not receiving effective management of pain from your prescription pain medication, talk to your health care provider. Similarly, if you are taking a prescription pain medication long-term, such as with a serious injury or disease, it is normal to build up a tolerance to your starting dose. This situation should be discussed with your health care provider honestly. Addiction to prescription pain medication is a need to continue to take the drug regardless of the harm it may be causing and is marked by withdrawal symptoms whenever the medication is stopped abruptly. Most student-athletes who take prescription pain medication exactly as prescribed do not develop addiction. In fact, some factors of addiction concern are predetermined. An individual with a previous addiction is more likely to become addicted to prescription pain medication, as are individuals with a family history of drug addiction.

It is important to discuss past experiences with pain medications, family history, and the progress of your pain management with your health care provider. If you are not finding relief from your prescribed regimen, your condition may have changed or worsened. These are the things your health care provider needs to know to find the right prescription and help you manage your pain. For these reasons, it is important to be honest with your health care provider.

THINK ABOUT IT

- ❑ What messages have you heard from your coach(es), family, and/or teammates regarding pain? Do you agree with their point of view?
- ❑ How would recovering from an injury affect your daily time schedule?
- ❑ Do you ever feel stressed out about the amount of pain medicine that you have to ingest? How else could you deal with your pain?

Playing Through Pain

Dealing with Performance Setbacks

When student-athletes experience setbacks during their training or competition due to illness, injury, or even just hitting a performance slump, they often have a very difficult time dealing with these conditions. For example, the best player on the basketball team may begin to miss even the simplest shots due to tendonitis in his or her shoulder, and athletes' emotions can be elevated by disappointment in themselves and/or fear that they have let down their coaches or been rejected by their teammates.

While emotions are part of the healing process, student-athletes should be careful not to let negative feelings overcome them. To maintain confidence and composure following an injury or setback, it is beneficial to recognize, regroup, and refocus your behavior. First, recognize that you may be off your game and that mistakes happen. Next, redirect your emotions of anger and frustration into positive energy, rather than dwelling only on your flaws. Finally, focus on the next play and set new goals for yourself. Following these steps, you can change how you react to mistakes and setbacks.

Every athlete has had at least one tough moment; for instance, a football player may have the wind knocked out of him by a hard tackle and as a result, he may fumble the football. He is left lying breathless on the field from the impact of the hit. The player feels devastated as the athletic trainer runs onto the field to assess if he is hurt, and the crowd's cheers fall silent. In this scenario, the player feels physically hurt, embarrassed, and emotionally upset. He must remember, however, that he can benefit from thinking more positively as opposed to giving up. To overcome his mistake and pain, he should recognize his error, take a few moments on the sidelines to catch his breath, regain composure, and refocus his efforts on running the next play pattern. It is pointless for him to dwell on his error. Additionally, it is not uncommon for athletes to feel angry after making a mistake. In this case, the player may be upset with himself for dropping the ball, feel anger at his teammates for not blocking, and/or be annoyed with his opponent for making an aggressive tackle. Negative feelings will not change what happened, so he should redirect his feelings in a positive way by visualizing that he will hold onto the ball during the next play. In all, student-athletes who are able to recognize setbacks, learn from their mistakes, and regroup with a positive attitude will be successful both on and off the field.

Teammates play an important role in the healing process, and student-athletes should not have to deal with setbacks by themselves. Players who support each other often develop cohesion and form true bonds by pulling together to overcome obstacles. A word of encouragement or a sign of confidence from a teammate can help a player recover from a performance or emotional slump. In the competitive world of sports, coaches scold and bench players for making mistakes, thus it is natural that a student-athlete's confidence is fragile. In all, as a player on a team, it is important to provide support and reassurance to your fellow teammates with either verbal or nonverbal reinforcement, such as a word of encouragement or a pat on the back.

Coping with Injury

Sports can improve student-athletes' physical condition, self-esteem, and attitudes, but being physically active can also cause damage to their bodies. Strains, broken bones, cuts, sprains, and bruises are the downside to competing in sports. When you are injured it is not only painful, but also very stressful and extremely time consuming, requiring rehabilitation, icing, heating, stretching, and practice. In addition to time constraints, dealing with an injury is also stressful, taking a toll on your ego and self-esteem. Perhaps for the first time in your athletic career, you are forced to sit on the sidelines rather than play. You may experience emotions such as resentment, denial, anger, and even depression. You must recognize that setbacks are hard to deal with, but they can be overcome. In all, overcoming an injury and regaining your confidence will make you a more focused and resilient student-athlete. Sometimes the hardest part of playing a sport is returning after an injury. Athletes typically have difficulty watching someone else play their position while they cannot participate.

Here are a few suggestions for coping with injuries. First, it is crucial that you accept that you have an injury, and acknowledge that you are the only one who can truly determine the outcome of your recovery. By taking on responsibility for your recovery process, you will find a greater sense of control and will progress quickly. A positive approach is more productive than dwelling on the past or blaming the injury on an outside factor. Next, you need to learn as much as possible about the cause, treatment, and prevention of your injury because if you do not fully understand your injury, it can cause fear or anxiety. Thus, you should ask a health care provider, trainer, coach, and/or therapist to clarify what you can do to heal quickly and completely. Write down and take with you the questions and answers recommended by the American Pain Association discussed earlier in this chapter. You need to be committed to overcoming your injury by going to treatments, working hard, and listening to your health care provider and/or athletic trainer to heal quickly.

If possible, ask another person to come with you to medical appointments. A parent, roommate, teammate, or coach are examples of people you might ask. This person's role is to listen and take notes with the purpose of helping you comply with the prescribed treatment and to provide you support during the process of healing and returning to the playing field.

You also want to maintain a positive mental state—for example, rather than thinking about your injury as a crisis, view it as a training challenge. In addition, set goals to keep yourself mentally motivated and positive. Work closely with your physical therapist, athletic trainer, or health care provider to set realistic goals and monitor your progress. For instance, you may be able to cross-train to maintain cardiovascular conditioning or strength. Ask your trainer, therapist, or physician to establish an alternative workout program. If you cannot run, perhaps you can cycle or swim. By working on flexibility, strength training, and nutritional health, you will be in great shape to reenter your sport once your injury has healed. Also, by monitoring your goals, you will notice small improvements in the rehabilitation of your injury.

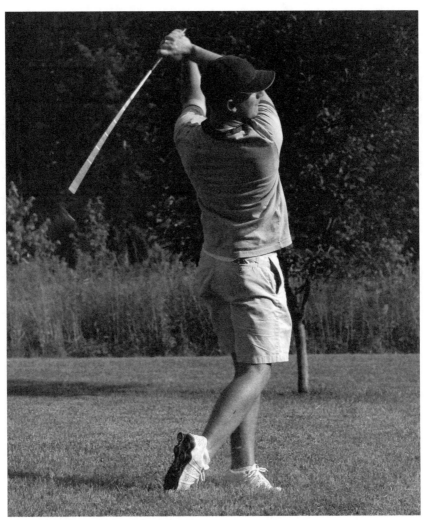

© Jeff Thrower (Web Thrower)/ShutterStock, Inc.

Additionally, because an injury can cause emotional strain, you should maintain contact with others to help you stay positive. Your teammates, friends, and coach can listen if you need to express anger, or they can offer advice or encouragement during the rehabilitation process. For many student-athletes, just knowing they do not have to face the injury alone can be comforting. Furthermore, try to remain a visible and active member of the team rather than isolating yourself. You should continue to attend practices and team meetings. Most important, you should not hesitate to cheer from the sidelines.

THINK ABOUT IT ✓

- ❏ Has there been a time in your athletic career where you suffered an injury and played through the pain? Did you tell the coach or athletic trainer about the injury? What made you able to keep playing despite the physical pain you were experiencing?

- ❏ Sometimes the physical pain of an injury can be easier to treat than the emotional pain. How can injuries be emotionally and mentally challenging for athletes to face?

- ❏ Reflect on a time when you were injured. What coping methods did you use to keep motivated and positive?

- ❏ Brainstorm a backup plan. If you were faced with a chronic injury, what goals could you set to redirect your energy when sports were not an option?

The majority of student-athletes have a tendency to try to speed up the recovery process, and they attempt to play before their body is fully healed. If you acknowledge your limits, know the facts, get support, and have patience, you can overcome an injury without long-term repercussions. In all, when student-athletes allow their bodies time to heal, set realistic goals, and remain positive, they can successfully overcome injury.

Preventing Pain and Injury

Personal Prevention Strategies

Injuries are often considered an inevitable part of sports. However, like other injuries, sports injuries are potentially avoidable. Probably since you started playing sports the importance of good preparation and injury prevention have been hallmarks of your training and performance. Adequate warm-up before participation, cooldowns after participation, correct stretching techniques (before, during, and after activities), core training, strength and aerobic exercises, and good nutrition all contribute to peak performance with few injuries. Less obvious and less discussed are extrinsic items that impact you as a player but are not under your control. Nevertheless you need to pay attention to them and be assertive to ensure your safety as well as the safety of your teammates. Equipment is primary among these items, especially footwear. Being aware of equipment also means knowing your playing surface and weather conditions. Even playing indoors, temperatures that are too hot or cold can affect your performance. Likewise, avoiding abrupt changes in training methods, efforts, and intensity, especially if you are struggling or performing below expectations, can prevent an injury that might sidetrack your season and performance.

Preventing injury is tied to you being assertive with other student-athletes about your needs and concerns. Frequently, student-athletes confuse being assertive with being aggressive. They are two different strategies. Trying to prevent personal injuries and problems as well as being part of a team requires you to hear the concerns and needs of your teammates and coaches and to voice your concerns and needs. The clearer you are able to be about your needs, the more likely they can be addressed, and then you can focus on performing well on the field as well as in the classroom and not waste time and energy.

Team and School Prevention Strategies

Prevention of pain and injuries also is part of the team's and school's responsibilities. Your role is to be assertive in making sure the team and school complies with these responsibilities. Think of yourself as an advocate fighting for your rights as a student-athlete. Request pre-participation medical examinations that can detect conditions that may predispose an athlete to injury. It is helpful to identify potential disabling conditions and musculoskeletal problems that need to be addressed prior to participation. Suggest rule changes and officiating procedures that encourage player safety and health. Work to improve equipment, playing surfaces, and conditions as well as to establish medical care at all practices and competitions. Prevention of sports injuries requires advocacy to ensure a proper environment for sports participation. You as a student-athlete know what concerns you and what will help you (as well as your teammates) be and compete injury and pain free.

Coaches, athletic trainers, teammates, and athletics directors are open to hearing your concerns. Schools have student-athlete advisory groups with representation from all teams at a school. Academic and athletic support programs often provide opportunities for student-athletes to make suggestions about how to improve conditions both on the playing field and in the classroom.

At times speaking up may seem to be more of a bother than it is worth. And it may well be, but it is important, particularly if your idea or comment contributes to a safe and healthy environment for student-athletes. Likewise, you may feel awkward speaking up. However, once again personal safety and injury prevention need to always be a priority for you, your team, and your school.

THINK ABOUT IT

- ❏ Reflect on how you prevent injuries. What are your personal strategies and routines to living injury and pain free?
- ❏ Brainstorm changes in the environment that would contribute to safer conditions during practice and competitions. Share them with your team manager and coach.

Career-Ending Injuries

Almost every athlete has to deal with setbacks, injuries, or failures during his or her athletic career. Setbacks are not necessarily a bad thing, as overcoming losses and challenges help athletes rise to the next level of competition. Unfortunately, not all setbacks can be overcome. In some instances, athletes suffer from conditions and injuries that can affect them for life. Some conditions, such as tendonitis or bursitis, can linger throughout an athlete's career, making it difficult for the athlete to perform at his or her best. Other injuries, such as those that require surgery or extensive rehabilitation, can be career ending. Handling an injury is extremely difficult for athletes, and therefore it is important to be prepared to deal with injury-related setbacks and have a backup plan if an unfortunate injury should occur.

Time after time, we hear about phenomenal athletes who become injured and whose athletic career is in jeopardy. Some of these athletes are able to return to their sport after rehabilitation, while others are never able to play again. For example, a promising twenty-year-old hockey star, Travis Roy, was a young hopeful in the world of professional hockey. After finally realizing his lifelong dream, an unexpected accident during a game changed his life. During his first collegiate game at Boston University, a freak accident drove Travis into the boards, and the accident left him with a cracked fourth vertebra causing him to be paralyzed from the neck down. While Travis could no longer play hockey, he remained positive and decided to speak out to the public about his life and dreams, touching the hearts of millions. In turn, he created an astonishing new life for himself. While he was never able to play hockey again, he remained active and involved in athletics. Travis's story includes drama, courage, determination, and the power of positive thinking, and he is a good example of a student-athlete who was forced to stop playing his sport but never gave up hope and his love of the game.

As athletes continuously push their bodies to the limits and coaches and trainers set high expectations on their performance, injuries have become more prevalent in competitive sports and are afflicting athletes at earlier ages. Almost every year, we hear in the media about the unfortunate football player collapsing from a heat stroke during training camp, or a wrestler in danger of dehydration. Situations like these force us to examine whether student-athletes are training too hard. Student-athletes must acknowledge their limitations as well as their abilities and work with coaches and trainers to make sure they are taking health and safety precautions during practice and competition.

It is important to recognize the psychological pain caused by injury and how the temporary or permanent loss of sport can have a significant effect on athletes. Whether an injury is career ending like the ones mentioned above or short term like a broken bone or a muscle tear, injuries can be devastating to student-athletes. Unless the psychological pain associated with injury is addressed, athletes face a hard road to recovery. The following are some tips for coping with career-ending injuries:

- Allow yourself to be upset. Feeling sad is an important part of the healing process. Injured athletes have a tendency to replay the incident in their mind and wish for a different outcome. Unfortunately, it is necessary to accept reality and acknowledge your loss.

- Try to stay positive. When positive, your attitude can speed up the healing process and lessen the emotional pain that you have to go through.

- Throughout the recovery process, set new goals and measure successes differently. An injury may mean that you will have to start at "square one" to rebuild your strength and endurance. Focus on taking small steps toward recovery and celebrate each success along the way.

- Brainstorm other ways to be involved in sports such as coaching, staying involved with the team, or trying a new activity. Let this be your motivation to heal.

- Seek support from your teammates and fight the urge to isolate yourself. Social support is crucial, and the worst thing for you to do when you're in a vulnerable state is to separate yourself from a support group.

- Seek the help of a professional therapist or counselor if you feel depressed for an extended period of time, lose interest in things you once enjoyed, notice that your sleep and eating patterns have changed, or have suicidal thoughts.

- Apply your skills to other areas of your life. As a student-athlete, you have developed many powerful assets, such as dedication, commitment, persistence, motivation, and the ability to manage setbacks. These attributes are sought by employers and can be transferred to other endeavors.

THINK ABOUT IT

- ❏ How would you respond to a teammate who does not deal well with losing?
- ❏ A teammate is feeling burned out because of the time commitment that it takes to play sports while balancing academics and social life. What advice would you give your teammate to make him or her feel less overwhelmed?
- ❏ Has stress from a bad practice or loss ever affected other areas of your life? What can you do to prevent setbacks in sports from causing you additional stress?

Student-Athletes and Technology

New technologies not only help us communicate and manage our time, but they also help us when we are injured. Advances in technology help us better diagnose and treat injury. For example, imaging devices such as CT scans and functional MRIs help doctors examine athletes who may have suffered broken bones, stress fractures, or tears. These devices are also used to evaluate athletes who have suffered head trauma and may be suffering from a concussion. Concussions are brain injuries that are fairly common in impact sports such as football and basketball. The symptoms of a concussion include headache, pressure, nausea, vomiting, dizziness, trouble balancing, blurred vision, passing out, being bothered by light or noise, feeling sluggish, confusion, memory problems, and difficulty paying attention. It is important that you tell your coach if you suspect you have a concussion or have taken a bump or blow to your head. If you have had a concussion, your brain needs time to heal. While your brain is still healing, you are much more likely to have a second concussion if you bump your head again. A second concussion can cause damage to your brain. It is important to rest until you get approval from a doctor or health care professional to return to play. Remember, it is much better to miss one game than the entire season.

Chapter Summary

Student-athletes have to learn how to deal with body aches, stiff joints, bruises, and strained muscles. Although these injuries are not particularly life-threatening or career ending, they are often viewed as badges of courage or "battle wounds." Whatever form of injury or pain student-athletes experience, it often raises a level of uncertainty and doubt because they are affected and cope in different ways. Thus, student-athletes' expectations of playing with a certain level of pain will vary individually because of pain level and pressures from teammates, coaches, and fans.

With injury come expectations that the athlete will do his or her best to keep performing, heal, and return to the sport because of a responsibility to themselves, teammates, coaches, and fans. Most student-athletes, however, realize it is critical that they learn to recover by pushing themselves enough, but not too hard, because the road to recovery will take a physical and emotional toll. You should acknowledge feelings of rejection, frustration, and anger common with pain and injury and deal with them just as much as the physical adjustments.

In all, as a student-athlete you probably are accustomed to the proverbial ice bag, ibuprofen, physical therapy, rehabilitation sessions, and even the possibility of a serious career-ending injury. However, you are an active member of your injury and pain management treatment team. Being prepared with answers to questions you know you are going to be asked as well as asking questions of your health care providers gets the best results. When you have an injury or are in pain, do not be shy and passive. Be assertive. Having a trusted person (family member, friend, coach) accompany you to your appointments and treatment to listen and ask questions is often helpful. Finally, you can be a leader and advocate in efforts to prevent injury and pain for yourself and teammates. It may be awkward to speak up about potential hazards and health-compromising situations, but make it a priority.

Your Thoughts

1. List what motivates you to continue playing even if you are experiencing pain. Please list separately the internal motivators (achieving personal goals, desire to win, and so on) and the external motivators (approval from coach, trophies, and so on).

2. Have you or a teammate ever been injured and worked to come back to the sport? What steps did you or your teammate have to take to accomplish this goal? What were the physical and emotional obstacles that you or your teammate had to overcome to return to playing the sport?

3. "No pain, no gain" versus "no pain, no brain." What is your personal attitude toward pain? Has there ever been a situation where you decided to risk injury to help your team win a single game, match, or competition? Did this one decision have a long-term effect on your health and performance in subsequent events?

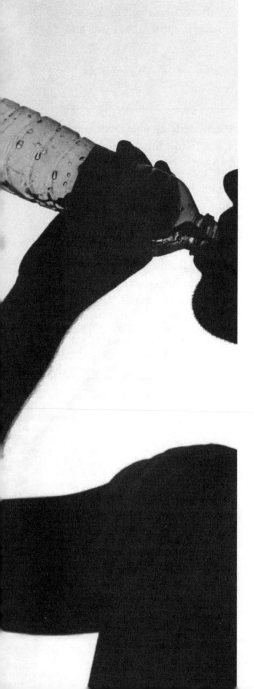

CHAPTER 5

Challenge #3: Sports Nutrition

Learning Objectives

After completing this chapter, you will be able to:

- *Identify the three sources of fuel for student-athletes and understand how nutrition affects athletic performance*

- *Understand the importance of vitamins and minerals*

- *Explain the USDA Food Guide Pyramid and dietary recommendations*

- *Read and understand food labels, evaluate a food journal, and develop a healthy, well-balanced meal plan*

- *Understand the effects, dangers, and warning signs of eating disorders such as anorexia and bulimia*

Student-Athletes Say:

- It is hard to eat healthy on a college campus with a meal plan, especially with my busy schedule. I usually just grab whatever is most convenient.

- I lose weight and gain it back all the time. I wish I knew how I could keep it off.

- I want to increase my performance this season; hopefully I can accomplish this by eating right and working out more.

- I heard about new diet pills that can help you lose up to five pounds. My friend told me they were dangerous to take while exercising and could potentially cause heart complications.

- Sometimes, when I get anxious or upset, I eat a lot of ice cream because it makes me feel better. After eating a lot of food, I feel depressed because I know I need to keep in shape for track.

- I noticed that TV and magazines today portray really skinny women as being active and fit. These women are not as muscular as me and it makes me mad and self-conscious.

For many college student-athletes, being at college is the first time in their lives they have the freedom to eat what they want, when they want. Juggling a full academic load, athletics, a new social life—and a college cafeteria with its smorgasbord of light and not-so-light foods—is a challenge. Fortunately, the skills for managing weight and sports nutrition are no secret. However, with so much information available about healthy choices, nutrition, and dieting, it is difficult for many student-athletes to choose the correct plan for their bodies and keep up with frequently changing information. Additionally, there are many fad diets available on the market, and many of them contradict each other.

As a student-athlete, it is important to eat well and maintain adequate energy levels. You need to educate yourself about the types of nutrients that are valuable for your body's performance. As a healthful eater you will resist disease and other stresses better than a person with poor dietary habits. Furthermore, well-maintained nutritional balance is critical during recovery from an injury; therefore, athletes need to select a diet that will keep them at the top of their game.

This chapter focuses on the information and skills you need for good nutrition. As a student-athlete, you need to make sure the decisions you make about what you eat maximize your performance. To get started, complete the Student-Athlete Challenge # 3: Sports Nutrition Self-Assessment in Box 5.1. Food and eating are part of your life in so many ways. Food fuels your

Box 5.1. Student-Athlete Challenge #3 *Sports Nutrition Self-Assessment*

Directions: Evaluate each statement on a scale of 1 to 5, from 1 being "never" to 5 being "almost always." For each statement evaluate if your behavior adds value (+), is neutral (0), or decreases value (–) of your student-athlete success in regards to your classes and sport.

Statement	Never				Almost Always	Value Added		
	1	2	3	4	5	+	0	–
1. I read food labels.	❏	❏	❏	❏	❏	❏	❏	❏
2. I eat a well-balanced diet.	❏	❏	❏	❏	❏	❏	❏	❏
3. I gain/lose weight easily.	❏	❏	❏	❏	❏	❏	❏	❏
4. I monitor my weight closely and weigh myself.	❏	❏	❏	❏	❏	❏	❏	❏
5. I keep a journal of my diet.	❏	❏	❏	❏	❏	❏	❏	❏
6. I eat even when I am not hungry.	❏	❏	❏	❏	❏	❏	❏	❏
7. I compare myself with people who are in magazines and on television.	❏	❏	❏	❏	❏	❏	❏	❏
8. I take vitamin supplements.	❏	❏	❏	❏	❏	❏	❏	❏
9. I feel that I am at a healthy weight.	❏	❏	❏	❏	❏	❏	❏	❏
10. I find it hard to find a healthy meal on campus.	❏	❏	❏	❏	❏	❏	❏	❏
11. I skip meals.	❏	❏	❏	❏	❏	❏	❏	❏
12. I am satisfied with my physical appearance.	❏	❏	❏	❏	❏	❏	❏	❏

athletic performance and gives you energy to attend class and study. At the same time the act of eating food is social and a big part of your life as a student-athlete. It is fun to hang out over a meal or snacks any time of day. Figuring out what works best for you is the challenge.

Whether you realize it or not, each time you sit down to a meal you bring to the table such factors as your own personal preferences, cultural traditions, and economic considerations. What you hear and see each day in the media plays an extremely powerful role in influencing our food choices and our knowledge of nutrition. These influences may exert an impact on your eating habits that is similar to hunger—the physiological need for food—and appetite—

the psychological desire for food, which may arise in response to the sight, smell, or thought of food even when you're not hungry.

> *Tennis was my life, and I took pride in the fact that I was always healthy and fit. I never thought I could be someone with an eating disorder, but I was wrong. It all started when I decided to skip sweets in order to shed a few pounds. I instantly felt lighter and had a lot more energy. My coach and teammates noticed the improvement in my performance and confidence level. I felt on top of the world.*
>
> *Later, I was reading a magazine article about how people who cut carbohydrates have an easier time getting thinner. As a gymnast, I had a lot of muscle, and I felt I was too bulky for a woman. I wanted to be leaner in appearance, so I decided that in addition to sweets, I would remove breads, pasta, and pretzels from my diet. I changed my diet so that the bulk of it was vegetables and meat. Once again, I lost weight and looked leaner.*
>
> *After I lost a few more pounds, my weight began to level off, but I still wanted to be thinner. I thought if I lost a few more pounds, I would be lighter on my feet and more graceful in matches, so I started skipping breakfast to cut out a few extra calories. At this point, I started to feel that my performance was suffering. I felt tired all the time and I had a hard time concentrating. I no longer had the energy to make it through practice, and often I became moody and upset. One practice, I even got lightheaded and dizzy to the point that I had to leave the court. My coach pulled me aside and asked what was wrong. When I told him, he explained to me that carbohydrates were essential for energy and endurance. He also told me there was a way to maintain or even lose weight without cutting out food groups. He encouraged me to speak with a counselor and nutritionist on campus.*

Sports nutrition is a subject that is forever changing. This chapter reflects the new information and many changes that have taken place in the field of sports nutrition in recent years. For student-athletes it provides the opportunity to develop practical skills in making decisions regarding their personal nutrition and health. The intent is for you to evaluate the facts for yourself and to apply what you learn in your own life.

Understanding Student-Athletes' Dietary Needs

Everyone's body needs food to provide energy and maintain function. Food supplies us with the energy that the body needs to replace worn or damaged cells and sustain the body. All food is composed of kilocalories and essential nutrients, which include vitamins, minerals, carbohydrates, proteins, fats, and water. Depending on the food, nutrients are found in various amounts; thus, it is important to remember that foods are not inherently "bad"—however, all foods are not created equal. Every food has different properties and different amounts of essential nutrients. For example, 12 ounces of soda has 160 kilocalories but virtually no nutrients, whereas 12 ounces of skim milk has approximately 85 kilocalories but also contains calcium, vitamin D, potassium, protein, and other nutrients. Thus, one cup of skim milk has a greater nutrient density than a cup of soda. Because the body needs nutrient-rich foods, it is important to consume foods that are full of nutrients, such as fruits and vegetables, which typically contain a higher percentage of nutrients per kilocalorie. In most cases, the deeper the vegetable color, the greater the nutrient content. For example, dark, leafy greens contain more calcium and vitamins than the whiter iceberg lettuce. The key to maintaining a healthful diet is consuming foods that enable you to take in all the necessary nutrients that your body needs to perform well without consuming more kilocalories than your body needs to function.

First, a kilocalorie is equal to one food calorie that you see on food labels on almost all packaged food products. A kilocalorie is the amount of energy it takes to raise one kilogram of water one degree centigrade at atmospheric pressure. Generally, when your body performs work by exercising or simply going about daily life, kilocalories are burned as your body is warming all of the water inside the body and releasing it as heat. Because all foods contain different amounts of kilocalories, certain foods are better sources of fuel than others. Just as a car can run with many different types of gasoline, our bodies can function on many different types of food. Cars get better gas mileage with premium gasoline, and similarly, the human body performs better with more nutrient-rich foods. Foods should never be labeled as good or bad; rather, they should be evaluated based on the amount and types of nutrients they provide. Foods with fewer nutrients are not the most efficient sources of fuel and may lead to negative health consequences. The challenge of keeping a healthy diet is finding the right balance of foods and eating the right quantity of kilocalories while consuming all the necessary proportions of nutrients.

MyPyramid (Figure 5.1) provides direction on how to balance your diet and monitor the number of calories you consume and the amounts of nutrients you need to perform at optimal levels. MyPyramid gives recommendations for how to balance your diet and get the proper amounts of each food group that the body needs. The Pyramid is divided into six food groups—grains, vegetables, fruits, oils, milk, and meat/beans. In addition, the Pyramid includes daily physical activity, which should be combined with a healthy, well-balanced diet to improve overall health and athletic performance. Each food group provides different nutrients to the body; therefore, you should include all the groups in your diet each day for optimal health.

Grains constitute the largest portion of the Pyramid. You should eat at least 6 ounces of grains each day. At least half of the grains you eat should be whole grains, which can be found in whole wheat bread, brown rice, and certain cereals. Next in the Food Pyramid are the vegetable and fruit groups. It is important to vary the fruits and vegetables in your diet, and eat at least 2.5 cups of vegetables and 2 cups of fruit each day. Each fruit and vegetable contains different vitamins and minerals, so you'll need to eat a variety. A trick to doing so, and in turn receiving a variety of nutrients, is to choose fruits and vegetables that are different colors. For example, eat green, leafy vegetables like spinach, orange vegetables like carrots, and red fruits like

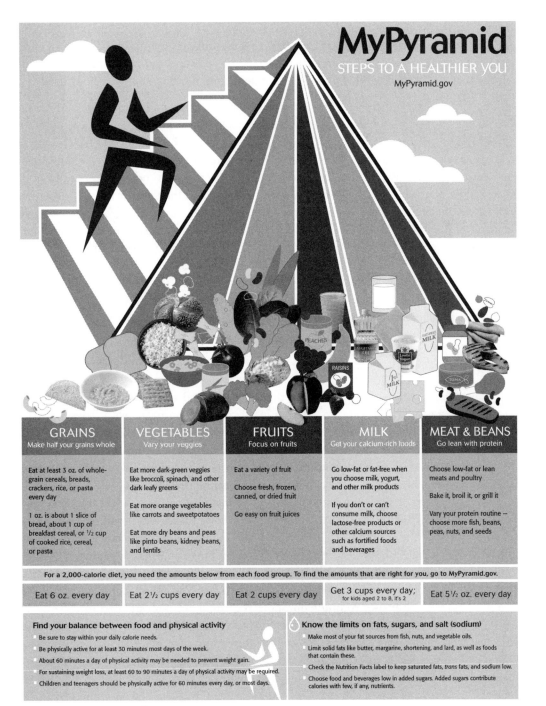

Figure 5.1 MyPyramid
Source: Courtesy of USDA

berries. The dairy group is another major food category within the Pyramid, and it is recommended that you eat or drink 3 cups each day. Low-fat milk, yogurt, and cheese are your best sources of dairy. Finally, it is also important to consume 5.5 ounces of meat or beans every day to make sure that you are getting all the fuel, protein, and nutrients that your body needs.

The first general principle behind eating a healthy diet and maintaining proper nutrition is balancing your diet. This means consuming foods from all the food groups each day. The more food groups eliminated from your diet, the less balanced your diet will be. One way to add balance to your diet is to include healthy snacks that contain at least three food groups. A good example is cheese, apple slices, and whole-wheat crackers. The crackers are from the bread and grain group, the cheese from the dairy group, and the apple from the fruit group. Because no one food contains every essential nutrient, eating a variety of foods can help you obtain all of the nutrients you need each day. For example, apples are a healthy snack, but if you eat an apple every day for breakfast, you are getting the exact same nutrients each day. Instead, you should try to consume other fruits such as bananas, oranges, and strawberries to maximize your nutrition by getting slightly different nutrients each day. A third underlying principle of good nutrition is portion control. The amount of each food we consume is important because whatever we consume and do not burn, we store as glycogen. People need to avoid foods full of empty calories typically found in sweets and candy because if you consume foods loaded with calories but do not have good nutrients, your body will receive a low level of nutrients.

Many student-athletes are pressed for time, have limited resources, have high levels of stress, and as a result, may resort to eating a lot of prepackaged meals with fewer nutrients. Some college students find it difficult to avoid bad eating habits like skipping meals or frequenting fast-food restaurants. Believe it or not, it is possible to eat a healthful diet even with limited time and resources. To help optimize your nutrition, you should be aware of a few tips for making wise food choices. For example, if you consume healthful foods, you will feel better, have more energy, cope better with stress, and perform better. Food is fuel and it affects all areas of our lives: academic, social, and athletic. Your body, mind, and mood may all suffer if you do not provide the correct amounts of the essential nutrients. For instance, think about a time where you skipped breakfast because you were running late in the morning. You probably had little energy and felt lightheaded or weak. Additionally, your may not have been able to focus or think as clearly in class. When you skip breakfast, you might also feel irritable and tired. This chapter will answer common questions regarding nutrition and performance as well as discuss healthy body weight and body image. These topics are especially important because weight is a very important issue for many college athletes who struggle to add a few pounds of muscle or to lose a few pounds before competitions. Whether you are trying to gain, lose, or maintain weight, there is a right and wrong way to approach it. This chapter will talk about some of the dangerous and healthy ways to manage weight, and also how to set healthy and realistic goals. Good nutrition plays a critical role in being a successful student-athlete.

THINK ABOUT IT ✔

- ❑ Name some strategies that can help you stick to a healthful eating plan.

- ❑ Would you approach friends, peers, or teammates to help you follow a healthful eating plan? How could you encourage your friends, peers, or teammates to follow a healthful eating plan or exercise schedule?

Nutrition in a Nutshell

Fuel Sources

Carbohydrates, proteins, and fats are not only essential nutrients, but also the only sources of fuel for the body. Each of these nutrients is required for the body to function properly and stay energized. Carbohydrates are an athlete's most important fuel source, and they should provide 60–70 percent of daily calories. They are found in a wide variety of foods such as breads, rice, fruits, vegetables, pastas, and cereals. The body converts the sugars and starches found in carbohydrates to energy (also known as glucose) and stores it in the liver and muscle tissues as glycogen. The two basic types of carbohydrates are simple and complex. Simple carbohydrates include foods that are high in sugar. They do not provide us with sustained energy; rather, they just give us a quick burst of fuel. Our bodies burn simple carbohydrates quickly and therefore they do not keep us feeling full and satisfied for as long as complex carbohydrates, which take longer to burn. Some complex carbohydrates are whole grains, brown rice, and foods with dietary fiber. Complex carbohydrates are especially important for athletes because they are the foundation of their energy. Athletes should be certain to eat carbohydrates for at least several days before exercise or competition in order to have glycogen-loaded muscles at the start of competition.

For instance, if your body runs out of carbohydrate fuel during exercise, it will burn fat and protein for energy; however, because fats and proteins are not the ideal source of fuel for exercise, your performance level will drop. To avoid running out of carbohydrates during competition or exercise, try to consume carbohydrates during bouts of exercise lasting more than an hour. This will help prevent fatigue and keep your body energized. Often athletes who compete in endurance competitions will consume energy drinks, such as Gatorade, which have carbohydrates (sugar) to maintain their optimal performance levels.

A second important source of fuel for the body is protein, which is composed of amino acids. Proteins are found in meats, fish, poultry, eggs, beans, nuts, and dairy products. Protein is essential to the diet because it helps the body build new tissue and repair muscles after exercise. Like carbohydrates, the two main types of proteins are complete and incomplete.

Complete proteins are found in animal products and contain all the necessary amino acids. Incomplete proteins, in contrast, do not contain every required amino acid, and therefore they must be combined with grains to get all essential amino acids. The average person's protein consumption should be 12–15 percent of their daily caloric intake. Because proteins are essential to building muscle, many athletes overestimate the amount of protein that they need in their diets. The amount of protein an athlete needs depends on his or her level of fitness, type of exercise, intensity, duration, and total caloric intake. Your body may use protein for energy if you exercise without eating more carbohydrates. A helpful way to calculate your recommended daily protein intake is to divide your weight by three. This number represents the number of grams of protein you should eat each day. The body does not store protein, and whatever is not used is stored as fat; therefore, it is important that you consume protein each day.

The body's final fuel source comes from fats. Fats have gotten a bad reputation in recent years, and are typically considered bad for the body. Regardless of rumors and current marketing, the body needs fat to function. Fats have several important roles in the body. They aid in absorption of vitamins A, D, E, and K, and they also protect organs. While fats are important, they can also be harmful because they are high in calories, and certain fats from animal products can increase cholesterol levels. Fats should be consumed in moderation and should constitute no more 20–30 percent of your caloric intake.

As stated previously, your body uses carbohydrates for fuel when you exercise. If your body uses up its glycogen supply and you continue to exercise, your body will burn fat for energy. Because fats are not as good a source of fuel as carbohydrates, exercise intensity and performance will suffer. The two main types of fats are saturated and unsaturated. Saturated fats are found in whole milk, butter, cheeses, and fried foods. These fats are harmful and should be limited in our diets because the body takes a long time to break down these fats. Unsaturated fats, in contrast, are better sources of fat because they actually increase your high-density lipoprotein (HDL), known as the healthy cholesterol in your body. In contrast, your body also has low-density lipoprotein (LDL), or the bad cholesterol, that can cause problems if you have too much of it in your blood. Unsaturated fat is typically found in nuts, olives, and canola oil.

Obviously, the proper amount of nutrition is important for student-athletes, but getting the correct nutrition on campus is not always easy. Take the example of two student-athletes going to the dining hall salad bar for lunch. The student-athletes' selections from a salad bar can make or break their healthful diets and either give them the boost they need or hinder their athletic performance. One student chooses iceberg lettuce, croutons, potato salad loaded with mayonnaise, bacon bits, and creamy dressing. The second student chooses dark, leafy greens, tomatoes, grated cheese, fresh fruit, tuna, and a low-fat salad dressing. In this scenario, the first student, through poor food choices, may have inadvertently consumed as many calories and fat as contained in a hamburger and fries. In all, student-athletes should put thought into their food selections. The choices you make at mealtime will affect your performance and determine how well fueled you are for competition.

Vitamins and Minerals

Many essential vitamins and minerals are needed in a healthful diet to help the body function properly. For example, vitamin B helps break down glucose, vitamin A is important for your joints, and folic acid is used in muscle tissue. Minerals, such as zinc, chromium, and potassium, are also critical elements of a healthy diet. These vitamins and minerals are especially important for athletes because they aid growth, carbohydrate metabolism, and cell growth, respectively.

Calcium and iron are two very important minerals in which many people are deficient, and these vitamins and minerals are especially important for athletes who put their bodies through vigorous training. In general, though, everyone should take special care to make sure that they get enough calcium and iron in their diets because they are critical for building strong bones and fighting fatigue; however, calcium is the most common mineral in the human body. Ninety-nine percent of the calcium in the body is found in the bones and teeth, with the remaining 1 percent found in the blood and soft tissues. If your blood levels of calcium are not maintained, your body will take calcium from the bones, lowering your bone mineral density and increasing your risk for osteoporosis. Therefore, adequate dietary calcium is a critical factor in maintaining a healthy skeleton. Males and females ingest calcium for storage only until the age of twenty-five, meaning that by the age of twenty-five, you have reached your peak bone density. The higher your bone density, the less likely you are to develop bone disease.

Although, most people think of milk when they hear the word *calcium*, you can get calcium from a variety of different foods, including cheese, yogurt, ice cream, canned fish, dark- green leafy vegetables, soft tofu, and fortified food items like orange juice or cereals. Even if you are eating a lot of calcium-containing foods, unfortunately, the body is not always efficient at absorbing this mineral. First, the body can only absorb 300–500 milligrams of calcium at one time. Since most people need 1,000–1,200 milligrams a day, they should consume three separate servings of calcium during the day to make sure they are actually absorbing the recommended amount. People who are concerned that they are not getting enough calcium in their diets should consider taking a calcium supplement. It is important to find a supplement that also contains vitamin D because it helps the body absorb calcium and deposit the calcium into the bones. The best food sources of vitamin D are fortified milk products and fatty ocean fish. Without enough vitamin D, you can develop weak or brittle bones, which can lead to rickets (soft bones) or osteoporosis (weak, brittle bones). Fatty fish, like salmon and mackerel, and cod liver oil are good sources of vitamin D. Vitamin D is one of the only things the body can synthesize or make on its own. The body synthesizes vitamin D when exposed to sunlight for thirty to sixty minutes. If you are exposed to sunlight on your skin two to three times per week, you can actually absorb all the vitamin D you need.

A second important mineral that is often lacking in men and women's diets is iron. The most important function of iron in the body is to carry oxygen in the red blood cells to the muscles. People without enough iron in their diets and who are deficient in this mineral become

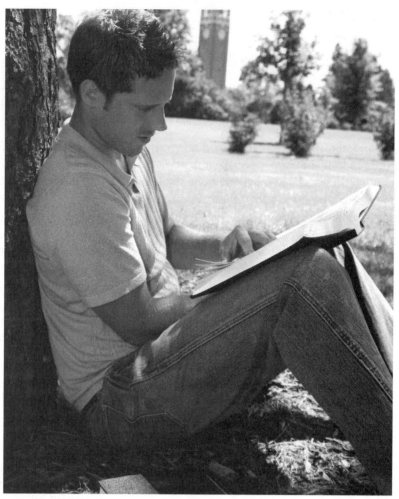

© Dana Bartekoske/ShutterStock, Inc.

anemic. Anemia can occur when there are not enough red blood cells, or when the cells are deficient and the exchange of oxygen and carbon dioxide between the blood and cell tissue is limited. Anyone is at risk for anemia, but most commonly vegetarians, female athletes, and runners are at greatest risk. Female athletes have a greater risk of becoming anemic because excessive sweating and menstruation increase the body's demand for iron. Runners in particular are at increased risk for becoming anemic because the impact on the body causes an increased loss of iron. Runners may also break blood vessels in their legs from the impact, which further increases their need for iron. Everyone should look for signs that they are not getting enough iron. Symptoms of anemia include pale skin color, fatigue, weakness, irritability, dizziness, shortness of breath, headache, sore tongue, brittle nails, decreased appetite, cracks in the side of the mouth, susceptibility to infection, and leg cramps while climbing stairs. If you are deficient in iron, you can modify your diet to get back on track. Iron is found in many foods that we eat. The two types of iron are heme and non-heme iron. Heme iron is found in animal sources, such as lean red meats, and 20 percent of the heme iron ingested is absorbed by the body. Non-heme iron, in contrast, is found in foods such as spinach, lentils, beans, iron-fortified cereals, chickpeas, almonds, apricots, and raisins. Unlike heme irons, only 3–8 percent of the iron found in plant foods is able to be absorbed. You can do a few things to increase iron absorption. One thing is to eat small amounts of heme iron coupled with larger amounts of non-heme iron, which will increase the absorption of the non-heme iron. Adequate vitamin C also increases absorption of iron. Vitamin C is found in kiwi fruits, green peppers, citrus fruits, strawberries, tomatoes, broccoli, and cantaloupe.

Typically, most female athletes are not aware of the amounts of iron that they must consume, 15–18 milligrams, in their diets to replenish their bodies' supply. Many athletes, particularly those who participate in distance or endurance events, eat diets that are high in carbohydrates and low in fat. It is important for female athletes to find sources of carbohydrates that are fortified with vitamins and minerals, particularly iron, so they can avoid vitamin and mineral deficiencies such as anemia. Look for fortified cereals, breads, and pasta to maintain peak athletic performance and a nutritious diet.

Hydration

Water makes up 50–75 percent of your total body weight. Water helps transport nutrients in the body, cleanses the body of waste, lubricates joints, serves as a shock absorber, helps maintain body temperature, and prevents dehydration. Water intake from drinks and food must equal water output from urine, colon, lungs, and skin. The average sedentary adult needs eight to twelve cups of water a day. Several factors, such as a high-protein or high-fiber diet, exercise, environment (e.g., extreme heat), certain medications, and illness increase the amount of water our bodies need. Dehydration is more common than most people think. Symptoms of dehydration include fatigue, dizziness, headaches, constipation, delirium, muscle cramps, and impaired athletic performance. Humans have a very poorly regulated thirst mechanism; therefore, if you are thirsty, chances are you are already dehydrated. The best way to monitor your own hydration status is to check the frequency and color of your urine. It may sound unpleasant, but the darker your urine is the more dehydrated you are (unless you are ingesting excessive vitamins, which can also make your urine brighter). When your urine is light in color, your body is better hydrated. Another way to make sure that you are getting enough water is to weigh yourself before and after exercise. You may be surprised to see how much weight we actually lose during one workout session. People can lose three pounds or more in a single session due to perspiration (water lost when you exercise).

THINK ABOUT IT ✓

❑ Eating a healthy and well-rounded diet takes time and consideration. Brainstorm some things you can do to make your diet realistic (e.g., preplanning meals, making lists for the grocery store).

❑ Eating out with friends or teammates does not always allow for the best diet. List some ways you can make healthy food choices, even when eating out.

❑ List some ways in which you could improve your current diet. Maybe it is only a matter of drinking more water or adding more protein. Which areas of your diet can be improved daily to help you be healthier?

Proper hydration is critical for student-athletes because all the training and hard work in the world will not help you in a tough competition unless your body is adequately hydrated. For example, during preseason soccer camp, players often have up to three practices a day. In late August, when it is hot and humid, the players have to be very cautious to maintain their body fluid levels. Dehydration will cause athletes to become fatigued and may even cause muscle cramps. Ideally, you should schedule drink breaks throughout your day. Two hours before practice, you should consume about two cups of water, and thirty minutes before practice you should consume another cup. During practice, you should take small water breaks every fifteen to twenty minutes. Finally, after practice, it is important to replace all fluids that were lost during the activity. A general rule is to drink two cups per every pound of water you lose. The key to making it through a long day of grueling training is to head off dehydration and never let your body fall below the recommended level of hydration.

An Athlete's Body

Finding Your Healthy Weight

College is a time when many males and females tend to put on a few extra pounds due to new eating patterns. Losing weight may become an important issue for some students, and it is important to know how to lose and maintain weight loss safely.

To begin, it is important to know what is a healthy weight for you and how to set realistic goals for yourself. People rely on two different measures to find their ideal body weight. The first body weight assessment is known as the Hamwi equation. The Hamwi equation factors in sex and height to determine a healthy weight. For example, five-foot-tall males should weigh 106 pounds (plus or minus 10 pounds). For each additional inch, males should add another six pounds to determine their ideal weight. In contrast, five-foot-tall females should weigh 100 pounds and should add an additional five pounds for each inch over five feet. The Hamwi equation accounts for body frame by stating that individuals with a small build should subtract 10 percent, while people with a large frame should add 10 percent to their score. For example, a five-foot-ten male should weigh 106 + (6 × 10 inches) or 166 pounds +/− 10 percent. This equation has limitations, especially when being used by student-athletes. Muscular people will weigh more than their ideal body weight because muscle weighs more than fat.

Another method used to assess body weight is the body mass index (BMI). The BMI is a formula that identifies whether an individual falls within a healthy weight for their height (Figure 5.2). The formula is as follows:

Weight in kilograms / Height in meters squared

BMI	19	20	21	22	23	24	25	26	27	28	29	30	31	32	33	34	35
Height							**Weight in Pounds**										
4'10"	91	96	100	105	110	115	119	124	129	134	138	143	148	153	158	162	167
4'11"	94	99	104	109	114	119	124	128	133	138	143	148	153	158	163	168	173
5'	97	102	107	112	118	123	128	133	138	143	148	153	158	163	158	174	179
5'1"	100	106	111	116	122	127	132	137	143	148	153	158	164	169	174	180	185
5'2"	104	109	115	120	126	131	136	142	147	153	158	164	169	175	180	186	191
5'3"	107	113	118	124	130	135	141	146	152	158	163	169	175	180	186	191	197
5'4"	110	116	122	128	134	140	145	151	157	163	169	174	180	186	192	197	204
5'5"	114	120	126	132	138	144	150	156	162	168	174	180	186	192	198	204	210
5'6"	118	124	130	136	142	148	155	161	167	173	179	186	192	198	204	210	216
5'7"	121	127	134	140	146	153	159	166	172	178	185	191	198	204	211	217	223
5'8"	125	131	138	144	151	158	164	171	177	184	190	197	203	210	216	223	230
5'9"	128	135	142	149	155	162	169	176	182	189	196	203	209	216	223	230	236
5'10"	132	139	146	153	160	167	174	181	188	195	202	209	216	222	229	236	243
5'11"	136	143	150	157	165	172	179	186	193	200	208	215	222	229	236	243	250
6'	140	147	154	162	169	177	184	191	199	206	213	221	228	235	242	250	258
6'1"	144	151	159	166	174	182	189	197	204	212	219	227	235	242	250	257	265
6'2"	148	155	163	171	179	186	194	202	210	218	225	233	241	249	256	264	272
6'3"	152	160	168	176	184	192	200	208	216	224	232	240	248	256	264	272	279
	Healthy Weight						**Overweight**					**Obese**					

Locate the height of interest in the leftmost column and read across the row for that height to the weight of interest. Follow the column of the weight up to the top row that lists the BMI. BMI of 19 to 24 is the healthy weight range, BMI of 25 to 29 is the overweight range, and BMI of 30 and above is in the obese range. Due to rounding, these ranges vary slightly from the NHLBI values.

Figure 5.2 Body Mass Index According to Weight and Height
Source: Reproduced from U.S. Departments of Agriculture and Health and Human Services. Dietary Guidelines for Americans, Sixth edition. Washington, D.C.: U.S. Government Printing Office, 2005.

Like the Hamwi equation, BMI also has limitations because it does not account for the amount of muscle that trained student-athletes possess. Using these weight measures, muscular student-athletes are often classified as being overweight because muscle weighs more than fat. Thus, athletes should use a different measure to evaluate their weight rather than relying on numbers derived from height and weight equations. Athletes should use body composition as their guide. For example, they can measure their percentage of body fat using skinfold measures or electronic body fat analyzer scales—bioelectrical impedance analysis. These techniques are better for evaluating people with muscular builds. These devices measure the percentage of your body that is fat and allows you to differentiate between lean muscle mass and fat. Women should have a body fat percentage between 20 and 30 percent, while males should be in the range of 12 to 20 percent.

Now that you understand how to evaluate your current body weight, you may feel that you need to lose or gain weight. It is critical when trying to gain or lose weight to remember the energy balance equation. In short, weight gain occurs when energy in food consumption is greater than energy output. Weight loss occurs when energy expenditure is greater than energy consumption. There are three components to energy expenditure that control how much energy a person burns. The components are resting metabolic rate, thermic effect, and physical activity (see Figure 5.3).

Metabolic rate is the energy required to keep the body functioning. Your resting metabolism or metabolic rate accounts for about 60–70% of your daily caloric expenditure. The second component is the thermic effect, which is the energy spent digesting and processing food. The thermic effect accounts for only 10 percent of your energy expenditure. The third component, which you can control, is physical activity. The more you exercise and engage in physical activity, the more energy you will use. Physical activity accounts for 20–30% of your energy expenditure. The key to successful weight loss is to unbalance the energy equation by decreasing caloric intake and increasing caloric expenditure through exercise. To see a change in body

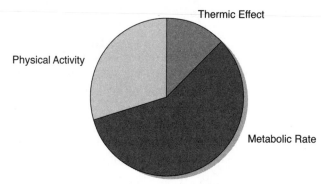

Figure 5.3 Three Components of Energy Expenditure

weight, you must offset the energy balance equation by 3,500 calories. This means that to lose one pound of fat, you must burn 3,500 calories. Achieving a 3,500-calorie deficit can be done healthfully by cutting 250 calories from your diet each day and adding twenty minutes of physical activity. Diet and exercise combined yield better results than diet or exercise alone. A healthy, energy-controlled diet incorporated with regular physical activity has been shown to be the most effective way to sustain weight loss.

A common error made by dieters is underestimating their caloric consumption while overestimating their calorie burn from physical activity. For example, the average person who eats a bagel that contains about 300 calories for breakfast will have to walk or run approximately three miles to burn the kilocalories he or she consumed. What if the person adds two tablespoons of cream cheese and jelly to their bagel? This would add an additional 150 calories. Now that person would have to walk or run an additional 1.5 miles just to burn off the bagel's toppings! To avoid dieting pitfalls associated with underestimating food consumption, learn to read and understand food labels and watch portion sizes. In all, you need to pay attention to calories, fat, sodium, and, most important, serving size.

Another common mistake made by people trying to lose weight is to cut their calories to extreme levels. It is important that you always eat at least 1,200 kilocalories per day. This is the amount needed to sustain your body's functions. Eating less then 1,200 calories a day will typically make you gain weight in the long run. When you eat less than 1,200 calories a day your body begins to think that it is starving, and the body will begin to store calories and fat because it needs all it can get to maintain homeostasis or life. As a result, your body learns how to run efficiently without burning as many carbohydrates or calories and your metabolism slows down in order to maintain internal functions.

Eating regularly and setting realistic goals are two effective ways to lose weight and maintain a healthy diet. First, if you eat regularly, you should eat breakfast and avoid skipping meals. It is not uncommon for student-athletes to get up in the morning and rush out the door without breakfast. It may seem like an easy way to cut down on calories; however, eating breakfast actually helps you lose weight because people who skip breakfast are more likely to overeat at lunch or grab an unhealthy calorie-packed snack. In all, you should try to avoid skipping meals, especially breakfast, because eating small frequent meals will help you maintain your metabolism and deter you from overeating.

Another tip is to set realistic goals. Setting realistic goals is not always easy for student-athletes, who are often in search of quick results. Much like training for a competition, losing or gaining weight takes time, and setting realistic goals is critical to success. A realistic goal includes trying to gain or lose no more than 10 percent of your current body weight. Also, student-athletes must give themselves adequate time to achieve their weight gain or loss goals. It is unrealistic and unhealthy to try to gain or lose more than one to two pounds per week.

Losing weight at a slow, steady pace has been linked to sustained weight loss. For example, a football player who weighs 200 pounds and wants to lose 15 pounds before the first game of the season can start a diet and exercise program three months before the season begins. He can try to lose one to two pounds per week by reducing his daily caloric intake and increasing his workout. Setting realistic goals will help him stay on track and not become frustrated with minor setbacks. By losing the weight slowly, he is more likely to keep the weight off during the whole season while keeping his energy levels up and performing well. Here are a few tips for reducing fat and calories in your diet:

- Choose foods that are baked or broiled rather than fried.

- Monitor serving sizes—i.e., avoid things like jumbo muffins, super-sized fries, or all-you-can-eat buffets.

- Stay away from snack foods that have "partially hydrogenated" or "hydrogenated" vegetable oil in the ingredient list. This is a manmade saturated fat that is hard for the body to break down.

- Try skim or 1 percent milk rather than whole milk.

- When eating meat, look for lean meats and trim excess fat.

- Choose healthful toppings on pizza, such as mushrooms or peppers, rather than sausage.

- Use fat-free or low-fat salad dressings to cut calories from the salad bar.

Disordered Eating

For some people, food is an obsession and can be associated with lifelong feelings of guilt and shame. Over 12 million Americans suffer from eating disorders, and symptoms include preoccupation with food, weight, and body image. Furthermore, eating disorders are one of the most prevalent psychiatric problems for women and girls. Less than a third of individuals with eating disorders receive treatment. Eating disorders produce symptoms for only 40–60 percent of patients; therefore, disordered eating poses a very serious health concern. Eating disorders can alter physiologic functioning, thinking, self-concept, relationships, and values. These disorders also have been shown to result in subjective distress and functional impairment, as well as hospitalization, suicide attempts, and even death.

The three most common eating disorders in the United States are anorexia nervosa, bulimia nervosa, and binge eating disorder. Anorexia nervosa is an eating disorder where people literally starve themselves. Anorexics may be at a body weight below 85 percent of the normal weight for their height, yet they cannot see that they are dangerously underweight. Anorexics do not want to believe or realize that they are literally starving themselves to death. Food, body image, and weight may always be on their mind, and individuals often think they are fat or overweight when they are not. Anorexia is extremely dangerous and can have long-term health effects.

Bulimia nervosa is an eating disorder in which the individual often has less control than anorexia. Victims of bulimia nervosa usually have a negative self-image and struggle with their weight. They, too, are intensely afraid of getting fat; however, those with bulimia deal with the fear a bit differently. Instead of denying themselves food, they indulge to excess and consume large quantities of food in a short time, then eliminate calories by overexercising or purging. Some purging methods include self-induced vomiting, diet aids, or using excessive laxatives. Bulimia is often harder to detect than anorexia, because bulimics typically appear at a normal body weight, because even with purging, the individual will still absorb a percentage of the kilocalories they consumed. There is one major difference between bulimia nervosa and anorexia nervosa. Unlike the person with anorexia nervosa, the person with bulimia nervosa often realizes the behavior is abnormal and even dangerous.

A third common disorder is binge eating disorder. This eating disorder is similar to bulimia nervosa as it includes bingeing and overeating. Binge eating involves having intense episodes of uncontrolled eating, consuming thousands of kilocalories within a short time. Unlike a person with bulimia, the binge eater does not purge after the episode. This inability to stop overeating helps fuel guilt, anxiety, and obsession with food that supports the cycle of this disorder. People with binge eating disorder are typically overweight or obese.

Eating disorders are long-term illnesses that can produce severe medical and psychological consequences. Anorexia can cause an irregular heartbeat, low blood pressure, lightheadedness, and fainting spells. It can lead to a thinning of the walls of the heart and, in females, amenorrhea. Amenorrhea is the loss of the menstrual cycle because there is not enough body fat to support it. This usually occurs when a female has 11 percent body fat or less. Prolonged amenorrhea leads to bone loss in females. Negative effects of bulimia nervosa include dehydration as well as tears in the esophagus and stomach. The stomach acid that comes up with the vomited food can cause tooth erosion, gum problems, and swelling of the salivary glands. Purging through the use of excessive laxatives can lead to life-long dependence, deficiencies of fat-soluble vitamins, and dehydration. Electrolyte imbalances from starvation or purging can cause muscle aches and cramps.

One source estimated that 20 percent or more of college students in America will experience anorexia nervosa or bulimia nervosa. Of these individuals, 90–95 percent are female; however, males are not safe from these disorders. The most common eating disorder among males is muscle dysmorphia. Muscle dysmorphia is an obsessive-compulsive disorder. It is sometimes referred to as "bigorexia," which is the opposite of anorexia nervosa. People with

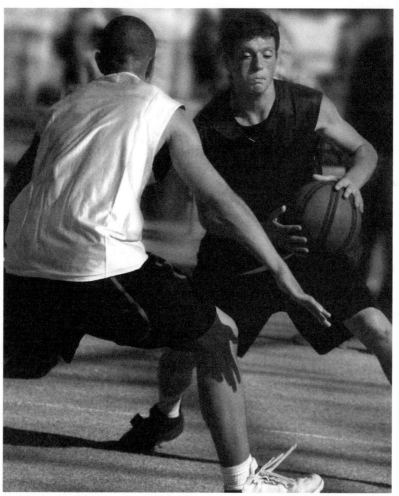

© Mirenska Olga/ShutterStock, Inc.

this disorder obsess about being too small and undeveloped; even when they have good muscle mass, they believe their muscles are insufficient. In an attempt to fix their perceived smallness, people with muscle dysmorphia lift weights, use resistance training, and exercise compulsively. These individuals may even take steroids or other muscle-building drugs to get bigger.

Eating disorders are becoming more and more prevalent on college campuses, and they are affecting student-athletes as well. Student-athletes are at risk for developing eating disorders because of the stress and emphasis they constantly place on their body and performance. For example, it is understandable that a female swimmer may feel a little self-conscious about her body. After all, she has to put on a swimsuit every day. When student-athletes become overwhelmed and feel exhausted by the pressures to look a certain way, problems may arise. For instance, the swimmer may constantly compare herself to her teammates in the locker room, and feel that she is not as thin or as muscular as the other girls. She may stress about every piece of food she puts in her mouth, and worry that she will look fatter than the other girls on her team. The swimmer may finish a long practice with her team and go off on her own to exercise more just because she is afraid that she didn't burn enough calories and she will gain weight. This student is exhibiting signs of an eating disorder and has a distorted body image. It is important that student-athletes are aware of different eating disorders and how they impact a player. Identifying disordered eating is the first step to overcoming the problem and the best way to prevent serious health consequences.

Eating disorders are also common in sports that place emphasis on athletes making weight requirements. For example, many wrestlers have disordered eating patterns. In this sport, where athletes must make a weight category to compete, they often go to extreme measures to lose weight quickly. They may starve themselves, dehydrate themselves, or even use laxatives to drop a few extra pounds before weigh-in. These methods can cause serious health problems over time.

Female Athlete Triad

Women have to be especially careful when it comes to healthy eating and balancing their bodies' needs. For women, restricting calories or disordered eating can have major consequences. Some female athletes who exercise intensely are at risk for a problem known as the female athlete triad. The female athlete triad is a combination of three conditions: disordered eating, amenorrhea (loss of menstruation), and osteoporosis. When a female athlete exercises intensely and does not eat enough calories, her weight falls and she may experience decreases in estrogen, the hormone that helps to regulate the menstrual cycle. As a result, menstruation may become irregular or stop altogether. Low estrogen levels coupled with inadequate nutrition cause females to lose bone density. As bone mass decreases, female athletes begin to develop osteopenia or osteoporosis. These conditions can ruin a female's athletic career by causing stress fractures and other injuries.

There are many suggestions as to why more females suffer from eating disorders than males. Some believe that the media places too much emphasis on beauty and has created unrealistic standards for body shape and size. Others suggest that the risk factors for developing eating disorders may be biological, genetic, and sociocultural. Research has shown that eating disorders often stem from body dissatisfaction, thin idolization, a skewed body perception, and low self-esteem. These disorders increase the risk for future onset of obesity, depressive disorder, anxiety disorders, substance abuse, and additional health problems. Therefore, it is crucial to look for the above warning signs if you or a friend are battling or developing an eating disorder. There is a way to treat and prevent these disorders, and numerous resources, including

Web sites, nutritionists, and counselors, can provide help and guidance. There is tremendous emphasis placed on student-athletes' bodies, and student-athletes are under enormous pressure to maintain a desired weight and perform at a specified level. This pressure makes disordered eating a problem among student-athletes. It is not uncommon for athletes to take their training and dieting too far. Many student-athletes think that they are enhancing their performance, but in reality rigid diets and overtraining can lead to long-term health problems. It is critical that student-athletes acknowledge their risk and pay close attention to maintaining a healthy and balanced diet.

THINK ABOUT IT

- ❑ Which method of measuring body weight is the most accurate for athletes? Why are some of the other scales used for evaluating ideal body weight flawed?

- ❑ One reason that many student-athletes do not eat healthful, balanced meals is lack of time. What are some ways you can try to fit healthful meals into your busy schedule?

- ❑ What are some of the signs that someone may be struggling with an eating disorder? Would you be able to differentiate between a teammate who was a very conscientious eater and one who had a disorder?

- ❑ If you thought your teammate was suffering from an eating disorder, how would you address that situation? Brainstorm some steps you could take to help.

PLUGGED IN TO SPORTS

Student-Athletes and Technology

Believe it or not, technology can even help us with our diet. Numerous Web sites provide healthy recipes and information on the nutritional content of our favorite foods. Some sites even have calorie calculators that allow you to enter the type and the amount of food you consume and see how many calories you are actually eating. Online tools are a great resource for student-athletes who are trying to fuel their bodies for competition while maintaining their weight and getting all the nutrients they need. A great way to track your diet and make sure you are eating a well-balanced diet and meeting all your daily requirements is to visit the Web site for the United States Department of Agriculture at http://www.mypyramid.gov. This site allows you to keep an online food journal, and it can help you to identify areas of strength and weakness within your diet.

Chapter Summary

Nutrition is a vital part of life! We eat for sustenance as well as pleasure. The extremes of eating too little or too much on a regular basis can be detrimental to your health, leading to eating disorders or obesity. Nutrition can also be used as an aid to increase performance. If you eat just before a workout or athletic event, it can hinder your performance. Similarly, if you consume too much fiber and liquid before an athletic event, it can also have you running to the bathroom instead of the starting line during a track meet. For optimal benefit, eat two to three hours prior to an event. You should snack on small food items closer to competition time and consume your main meal well in advance so your body is finished digesting and you have enough energy to perform without feeling hungry. Fat is also the hardest macronutrient to digest, so no matter what sport you play, a lower-fat meal is ideal prior to an event. You cannot perform your best without the right balance of foods and nutrients. For example, iron is important because deficiencies such as anemia can leave especially female athletes tired, weak, and short of breath. Furthermore, hydration is also a critical part of one's diet because water is considered one of the body's most essential nutrients. Most collegiate athletes typically consume unhealthful foods on a regular basis because it is more convenient, but healthful foods are also available. Remember the tips in this chapter to assist you with making better choices when eating out, because it is never too late to start eating healthier!

Your Thoughts

1. Do you notice that you eat certain foods when you experience different kinds of emotion or stress? For example, when you were younger, were you rewarded with food for doing something well? For two days, keep a food journal and write down your mood and emotions next to the food that you consumed. See if your mood affects what you eat.

2. Many student-athletes talk a lot about food and wanting to eat better. Why do you think it is so hard for student-athletes to change their eating habits?

3. Keep a food journal for two days. Write down the types of food you eat and the amount. Do you think people are more or less likely to make healthy food choices if they write down what they are eating and keep a food journal? Why?

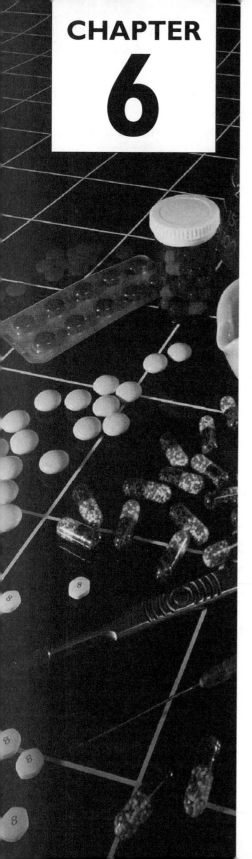

CHAPTER

6

Challenge #4: Performance Enhancers

Learning Objectives

After completing this chapter, you will be able to:

- *Define ergogenic aids and identify the five types*

- *Critically evaluate ergogenic aids and make healthy decisions regarding their use*

- *Evaluate eight common ergogenic aids according to whether they are effective, legal, and safe*

- *Discuss why athletes are tempted to use illegal ergogenic aids and the pressures that student-athletes face*

- *Understand the rules and regulations that govern the use of ergogenic aids in collegiate sports*

© Photos.com

Student-Athletes Say:

- One day a week, I have to do long runs where I run for a couple of hours. After about an hour, my body feels completely depleted. I carry a gel packet with me in order to give my body an extra boost when I start to feel fatigued.

- For many years, I have tried to increase my body mass by lifting weights, and I have had little success. My teammates suggested that I try creatine to increase my workouts and muscle size.

- I read that caffeine can help with performance and endurance, but my coach warned me that you can get hooked on it. Now I am worried that I drink too much of it.

- During high school, I won every race. I heard a rumor that some of my opponents in college were blood doping to improve their endurance. I wondered if this would help me to win again.

- My teammates use carbohydrate loading to prepare for events. I am nervous to try it because I don't know how it will affect my game.

- My best friend lost his scholarship when he failed our school's athletic department random drug test; that would never happen to me.

As a college student-athlete, you are under a lot of pressure to perform at an advanced level where competition is fierce. To keep up, student-athletes train hard and push their bodies to the limit. Often, student-athletes try ergogenic aids to enhance their performance. An ergogenic aid is defined as any substance, food, chemical, or training method that helps the body work harder and perform better. Athletes strive for the leading edge and many of them use ergogenic aids to improve their energy and performance. These aids can be as simple as a cup of coffee to give them a jolt before practice, or as extreme as injecting anabolic steroids directly into their muscles to gain extra muscle mass quickly before the start of the season.

It's easy to see why college student-athletes need to figure out how they are going to address ergogenic aids. Reading your favorite sports magazine, you are overwhelmed by the articles and advertisements detailing and promoting the attributes of a number of different types of ergogenic aids. Your local pharmacy, food market, and nutrition store have on their shelves many products that make claims to guarantee safe and effective ways to improve your performance. In contrast, the NCAA provides clear guidelines and regulations on the use of ergogenic aids. What is a college student-athlete to do?

This chapter focuses on the information you need to make a good decision about the role of ergogenic aids in your life as a college student-athlete. Probably for as long as you have been playing sports you have been using or know people who use aids to improve their athletic performance. As you complete Student-Athlete Challenge #4: Performance Enhancers Self-Assessment in Box 6.1, think about the range and type of aids that are available to you. Do you consider any aids safe, legal, and effective? Are there aids you believe are dangerous (i.e., unsafe and/or ineffective), even if they are legal and being used by people you know?

Ergogenic aids are common on college campuses and are often readily available to student-athletes. All student-athletes must decide for themselves if they are going to use aids to enhance their performance. As with anything, there are both negative and positive consequences to using ergogenic aids. Even those that are legal and safe, such as creatine, have their costs. One student-athlete describes his dilemma regarding the use of ergogenic aids:

> During high school, I had no problem keeping up with the other players on the track team. In college, I found that hours of hard work were no longer enough to stay ahead of the competition. Many of my teammates were taking pills to give them an advantage. One of my teammates told me that he used creatine to help get bigger and perform better. I wondered if I could get the same results.
>
> I began using creatine and got stronger over time. Unfortunately, my stomach was often upset, and I would often get muscle cramps after practice. Despite the minor aches, my shot put distances increased and my coach was impressed with my improvements. Creatine helped my game, but it was making me feel sick. I questioned whether winning was worth the pain.

As a college student-athlete who is serious about physical performance you are looking for an edge, maybe in the form of a legal, safe, and effective ergogenic aid to improve the parameters of your athletic performance and achievement. This chapter helps you consider your available options to find a performance enhancer that is legal, safe, and effective. Not only are there a tremendous variety of aids, but what works for one person may not necessarily provide the same benefits for another.

Understanding Ergogenic Aids

Throughout the year, athletes train almost every day and maintain rigid and rigorous schedules. Many athletes use ergogenic aids, which are techniques, devices, and substances that enhance performance, to sustain their intense training schedules. The majority of ergogenic aids used in athletics, such as dietary supplements and training techniques, are legal and acceptable. For instance, almost every athlete has had a caffeinated beverage; however, unlike caffeine, numerous ergogenic aids are illegal or have been banned by the NCAA, the Olympic committee, the National Football League, Major League Baseball, and other athletic organizations.

Box 6.1. Student-Athlete Challenge #4: *Performance Enhancers*
Self-Assessment

Directions: Evaluate each statement on a scale of 1 to 5, from 1 being "never" to 5 being "almost always." For each statement evaluate if your behavior adds value (+), is neutral (0), or decreases value (–) of your student-athlete success in regard to your classes and sport.

Statement	Never				Almost Always	Value Added		
	1	2	3	4	5	+	0	–
1. My teammates use performance-enhancing supplements.	❏	❏	❏	❏	❏	❏	❏	❏
2. I use caffeine to keep myself energized.	❏	❏	❏	❏	❏	❏	❏	❏
3. I use creatine to build muscle mass.	❏	❏	❏	❏	❏	❏	❏	❏
4. I use diet pills to try to lose a few extra pounds.	❏	❏	❏	❏	❏	❏	❏	❏
5. I look down on teammates who use performance-enhancing supplements.	❏	❏	❏	❏	❏	❏	❏	❏
6. I take vitamin supplements.	❏	❏	❏	❏	❏	❏	❏	❏
7. I condone the use of legal ergogenic aids (such as caffeine, amino acid supplements, and dietary supplements) in college sports.	❏	❏	❏	❏	❏	❏	❏	❏
8. One of my teammates failed a drug test.	❏	❏	❏	❏	❏	❏	❏	❏
9. I eat energy bars and drink sports drinks.	❏	❏	❏	❏	❏	❏	❏	❏
10. I feel pressure to use ergogenic aids to keep up with the competition.	❏	❏	❏	❏	❏	❏	❏	❏
11. Coaches and trainers give me advice on what supplements and performance-enhancing techniques that I should use.	❏	❏	❏	❏	❏	❏	❏	❏
12. I use ergogenic aids without knowing the side effects or consequences.	❏	❏	❏	❏	❏	❏	❏	❏

Five types of ergogenic aids are mechanical or biomechanical, psychological, pharmacological, physiological, and nutritional aids. Safe ergogenic aids include carbohydrate loading; proper nutrition; electrolyte solutions to replace lost fluids; and ritual preparations, such as prayer, positive imagery, meditation, visualization, and stress management. Some ergogenic aids can have harmful side effects. These are banned by sports-governing bodies because they are unsafe and unethical.

The activity in Box 6.2 will help you to reflect and identify to what extent and degree ergogenic aids are a part of your training routine. It will help you identify ergogenic aids and their impact on a student-athlete's body.

Before using ergogenic aids, you need to first evaluate their dietary requirements so you can understand how they will affect your body and what aid will be least harmful. For example, if you are considering using protein supplements to increase muscle mass, you must first evaluate the amounts of amino acids and complete proteins you already consume. If you decide to use a supplement, you must be aware of possible false claims, research or testing that was conducted, and physiological effects reported by the manufacturer. Any supplement that claims instant performance improvements without the assistance of hard work and training is a scam.

STUDENT REFLECTION

Box 6.2. How Do You Feel About the Use of Ergogenic Aids?

Have you ever experimented with ergogenic aids? Explain.

Which ergogenic aids have you tried?

Do you feel they work? If so, why?

Can you list one example of each of the following types of ergogenic aids?

- Mechanical or biomechanical
- Psychological
- Pharmacological
- Physiological
- Nutritional

Which type of ergogenic aid from the list above do you feel is the least harmful? Why?

Which type of ergogenic aid from the list above do you feel is the most harmful? Why?

THINK ABOUT IT ✔

- ❑ How might the use of an ergogenic aid affect your relationship with teammates/ opponents?
- ❑ List some common ergogenic aids you have heard about. Have you considered using any of them? Why or why not?

Eight Common Performance-Enhancing Aids

Carbohydrate Loading

Carbohydrate loading is a technique where athletes vary the amount of carbohydrates they consume in order to increase the amount of glycogen they can store in their muscles, thus enhancing performance and delaying fatigue. The technique is typically used by runners and cyclists and the process is completed over a period of six to eight days. First, an athlete will attempt to exhaust current stores of carbohydrates in his or her muscles through vigorous exercise. For the next few days, the athlete consumes minimal carbohydrates and continues to exercise in order to deplete the body's glycogen stores. Athletes often reduce the amount of carbohydrates they consume to 10 percent of their dietary intake in order to deplete the glucose in their muscles. At this point, the body will try to compensate for this muscle exhaustion by storing greater reserves of glycogen in the muscle. After several days of low carbohydrate consumption, the body will utilize glycogen stores. When the athlete resumes eating carbohydrates, the body will respond by storing more glycogen than normal. Therefore, prior to competition, the athlete increases carbohydrate consumption significantly and reduces his or her physical activity, escalating energy glucose stores in the muscle. Typically, three days before competition, the athlete will consume nearly 80 percent carbohydrates and reduce the training load. The theory is that the body will overcompensate and store extra energy (glycogen) in the muscle. Student-athletes must be cautious when carbohydrate loading. For instance, reducing carbohydrate intake too greatly can be dangerous because a healthy person's body needs at least 60 grams per day to maintain the function of several important internal systems. Also, athletes should be cautious not to overeat during the last few days of the carbohydrate loading process when they are consuming high amounts of carbohydrates. During carbohydrate loading, it is also important that the athlete consume more fluids than normal.

Furthermore, it is essential that athletes consume adequate protein, minerals, and vitamins. Thus, if you decide to engage in carbohydrate loading, try it in stages during your training months before your competitive session. In fact, many athletes will try a modified approach to carbohydrate loading, where they eat a low-carbohydrate diet for one day in an attempt to deplete their glycogen stores. Next, they consume a higher amount of carbohydrates just before competition. If athletes experience no adverse effects, they will extend the period of the low-carbohydrate diet to a maximum of three days. To track their bodies' reaction to carbohydrate loading, they should keep a detailed food and activity log. For example, a cross-country runner who is trying carbohydrate loading for the first time would choose to limit carbohydrate intake two days before competition. Next, the runner would work out in order to deplete as much of his or her glycogen stores as possible. Finally, the day before competition the athlete will eat a carbohydrate-rich diet. This student-athlete should feel energized for the competition event as the body should have maximum stores of glycogen.

Caffeine

Almost everyone drinks coffee in the morning to jump start their day, or has soda in the afternoon to get them through a long afternoon. When people become daily caffeine users, both their health and performance may suffer in ways they are not even aware of. For example, one of the biggest risks is that caffeine use disrupts sleep. Caffeine increases the length of time it takes to fall asleep and decreases total sleep time. Some studies have shown that consuming even a moderate amount of caffeine early in the day can reduce the quality and quantity of that night's sleep, and it does not require someone consuming an energy drink right before bed for them to experience the effects of caffeine. Disrupted sleep can pose a significant problem for college students because they may not get the recommended amount of sleep.

Many athletes use caffeine in coffee, tea, or pill form, believing that it will give their performance a boost; however, clinical studies suggest that there is no obvious benefit for high-intensity workouts. Athletes often use caffeine because they hear it makes people feel less drowsy and reduces fatigue. Student-athletes use high doses of caffeine to boost attention and concentration, prolong exercise, improve aerobic capacity, and control their weight. While caffeine may give your body a boost, it may also make you less steady on your feet and cause shaky hand movements. At high dosages, caffeine can cause anxiety, nervousness, increased blood pressure, disordered eating, insomnia, and an irregular heart rate. It also disrupts energy supply, fluid levels, and availability of nutrients in the bloodstream, thus hurting the consistency of your performance rather than enhancing it. Even though caffeine is not illegal, excessive use can get you banned from competition. Coffee-loving athletes should be aware that they could be disqualified from competition if they go over the threshold of 12–15 mg per ml.

Student-athletes need to be careful about their caffeine consumption because sleep and rest are essential for repairing muscle tissue and performing optimally. However, most students who drink caffeine daily will build up a tolerance to the substance. They will gradually need larger amounts to achieve the same effect, and over time they may feel dependent on caffeine to function normally. When it comes to chronic caffeine users, it is often difficult to separate the influence of the drug from the effect of not having the drug. In other words, they may think caffeine makes them feel and perform better, but in reality, caffeine inhibits them from feeling bad. Few nutritionists advise to avoid caffeine entirely, but they do advise people to consume it in moderation. Limiting caffeine use can be challenging because it is a common ingredient in many foods and drinks. To avoid becoming physically addicted to caffeine, athletes should not use more than 100 milligrams a day. This amount equals drinking one caffeinated soft drink or a small cup of coffee a day. For athletes who find that recommendation unrealistic, nutritionists advise that they keep their daily intake under 300–400 milligrams a day. Keeping consumption under 400 milligrams will reduce the likelihood of side effects such as sleeplessness, restlessness, and digestive disturbance.

Furthermore, caffeine has physiological effects on the body. Coffee and colas are high in phosphorus, and the body requires a certain phosphorus-to-calcium ratio. If your phosphorus intake is high, and you do not consume enough calcium, your body will take calcium stores from your bones, which will eventually make your bones weak and susceptible to injury; therefore, daily consumption of coffee and colas deprives the body of calcium. Most athletes do not understand that calcium in their diets is critical, and when they exceed normal caffeine consumption the effect on their body can be disastrous. When daily calcium intake does not outweigh their use of coffee and colas, they experience negative reactions. The first negative reaction can be the increased production of stomach acid that can lead to an upset stomach or acid reflux. Second, while caffeine is no longer believed to be a diuretic, most caffeinated beverages are not particularly good sources of hydration. For example, in endurance sports, caffeine can enhance performance; however, it is important to understand the effects that caffeine has on the body's hydration levels because sufficient hydration is critical for a successful athletic performance. In all, if athletes replace water or sport drinks in their diets with caffeinated beverages, their chance of dehydration will increase.

Finally, caffeine consumption should be monitored because heavy consumption can produce psychological effects, such as anxiety. For instance, the coffee retailer Starbucks reports that its 16-ounce coffee contains 400 milligrams of caffeine, which is the exact amount researchers administered to participants during a research study to induce anxiety. Student-athletes already experience a lot of anxiety; thus they must be careful not to add any unnecessarily. For example, it is normal for a student-athlete to have an exam looming, a paper due, and a big game all at the same time, and it is not uncommon for a student-athlete to drink a mug or two of coffee or an energy drink to make it through the day. Student-athletes must be careful not to overdo it because they do not need the added feelings of stress and anxiety. Most students do not realize that consuming too much caffeine will hinder their mood and feelings rather than improving their productiveness.

Steroids

Anabolic steroids are synthetic drugs that artificially increase testosterone and help build body tissue. Steroids were initially created for medical purposes, but today they are often used in high doses by athletes eager to improve performance and gain strength quickly. Athletes abuse steroids by taking 100 times the dose prescribed for medical use. Anabolic steroids come in a variety of forms, including pills, creams, injections, and gels. The most commonly used steroids include Anadrol, Oxandrin, Winstrol, Durabolin, and Equipoise.

There is tremendous controversy regarding steroid usage in professional sports because they are considered banned substances. While steroids have been proven to increase strength and anaerobic activity, they cause a plethora of side effects and health risks that can prove fatal.

Steroid usage is increasing among adolescents, which may be shocking information for many adults. It is estimated that almost 3 percent of all eighth through twelfth graders have taken some sort of steroid. In addition, also estimated is that hundreds of thousands of adults eighteen and older have used steroids. Use and abuse are higher among men than women. Box 6.3 lists some of the most common side effects associated with steroid use.

STUDENT REFLECTION

Box 6.3. What Are Possible Health Consequences of Steroid Usage?

Musculoskeletal
- Tendon rupture
- Premature closing of the growth plates on the long bones in adolescents

Cardiovascular
- Heart attacks
- Enlargement of left ventricle
- Increased blood pressure

Infections with Needle Usage
- Hepatitis
- AIDS

General Health
- Liver/kidney cancer tumors
- Fluid/water retention
- Suppressed immunity
- Headaches, nausea
- Cholesterol (increases LDL, decreases HDL)
- Acne/rashes

Hormonal and Sexual Side Effects

Men
- Infertility—low sperm count
- Testicular atrophy
- Decreased testosterone
- Lowered sperm count
- Variable sex drive

Women
- Increased facial/body hair
- Deepening voice
- Menstrual irregularity or cessation
- Decrease in breast tissue

Psychiatric Effects
- Homicidal rage
- Mood swings/aggressiveness/irritability
- Nervous tension
- Mania and/or depression

As in the vignette at the beginning of this chapter, when student-athletes enter collegiate athletics, they are often surprised by the intensity of competition. Many student-athletes worry about keeping up and performing at an advanced level, and they are often tempted to try steroids to achieve a greater competitive advantage. Student-athletes should understand the health risks that are associated with steroid use before they find themselves in unhealthy or life-threatening situations, because if they are aware of the risks then the promised gains may seem far less appealing.

Creatine

Creatine is an ergogenic aid that is used to build muscle mass rapidly. Creatine supplementation aids those engaged in sports characterized by power and strength, such as football, track, weightlifting, and bodybuilding. Creatine can improve performance by enhancing actions that require quick bursts of energy or strength. While many athletes are using this dietary supplement and observing positive results, it is still important to remember that long-term effects of this substance are unknown. Similar to other "sports supplements," creatine claims to regulate muscle function and build work capacity, lean mass, and strength. Creatine's ergogenic value is due to its role in the creatine–kinase–phosphocreatine pathway in muscle tissue. A growing body of evidence indicates that this pathway is a conduit through which cellular energy is coordinated in muscle. Creatine supplementations, unlike other dietary aids or "body building" supplements, improve metabolic power and capacity by affecting muscles' energy.

Creatine has become commonly used; however, many people consume this supplement without even knowing the consequences or potential risks associated with this product. Creatine can quickly build muscle mass in most people, but there are side effects that are most recently being discovered by users. A few of the known short-term risks associated with creatine usage are muscle cramps, pulls, tears in tendons, and stomach distress. Most of the studies to date have observed creatine usage for short periods of time, generally about a month, thus no one really knows the long-term effects. Thus, student-athletes should be significantly concerned about taking this supplement. While short-term effects may be positive and have little consequence, there may be very painful and serious complications later in life. There is a need for more research to examine the effectiveness as well as the long-term health risks associated with creatine.

Many student-athletes, especially wrestlers and football players, use creatine to supplement their strength training programs. Taking creatine can help student-athletes increase lean muscle mass; however, it is important to remember that supplements such as creatine work only when used properly and combined with a healthy diet and rigorous training. Using a supplement such as creatine alone is not going to improve your performance.

Blood Doping

Blood doping is the method by which athletes increase the amount of red blood cells in their body in an attempt to improve aerobic performance. First, a person draws a unit of blood from the body and stores it. After three weeks, the body will completely replace the blood lost. The person next transfuses the blood back into the body. The result is extra red blood cells in the body. With more red blood cells present, extra oxygen is carried to the muscles, and this allows for heightened performance, particularly in endurance sports. The practice of blood doping is illegal in competitive sports because it gives athletes an unfair advantage.

Numerous risks are associated with this technique, and it is possible that blood doping can have unintended negative consequences. For example, a large infusion of red blood cells can cause an increased concentration of cells in the blood, thus increasing blood viscosity and

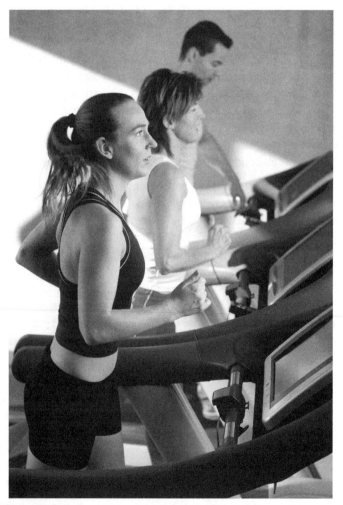

© Arne Trautmann/ShutterStock, Inc.

bringing about a decrease in cardiac output, blood flow velocity, and peripheral oxygen content. All of these consequences reduce the body's aerobic capacity. For instance, visualize the heart pumping blood the consistency of water through its arteries; now imagine that the heart is forced instead to pump blood the consistency of jelly. The heart has to work twice as hard to pump the dense matter through the arteries and veins. The human heart was not designed to pump this thickened blood throughout the body; doing so can lead to a multitude of problems such as phlebitis, septicemia, hyperviscosity syndrome, heart failure, bacterial infections, and potentially death. Furthermore, it is possible for those participating in blood doping to acquire diseases that can be contracted through blood transfusions and sharing needles, such as hepatitis, AIDS, and malaria.

One real-life example of blood doping consequences can be found in the story of the 1984 United States Olympic cycling team. American cycling teams had never fared well in the Olympic games, and in the 1984 Los Angeles games, the U.S. cycling team decided to try blood doping as a way to get an advantage on the competition. Initially, the results of using the substance were positive and the team won a U.S. cycling team record of nine medals. The negative consequences of blood doping resulted later, between the Olympic trials and the actual competition, when the Americans did not have adequate time to use their own blood for the transfusion. Instead, they used the blood of relatives and friends with similar blood types. Consequently, some of the cyclists received tainted blood, and a short time after the Olympic games those cyclists contracted a serious liver disease, hepatitis.

Therefore, the act of blood doping is a controversial issue, and whether or not blood doping is safe, effective, or ethical will be debated for years to come because of the new advances in science and sports medicine. Many present and future student-athletes will have to use their best judgment when the consequences of blood doping become an issue in their lives. Because blood doping is hard to detect, student-athletes may feel that their risk of being caught is minimal. Student-athletes must ask themselves if short-term performance enhancement outweighs the risks associated with the technique. They must also consider the ethical implications of trying a procedure such as this, which is proven to give an unfair advantage. Student-athletes who are desperate to enhance their endurance performance should consider altitude training, which can have physiological effects similar to that of blood doping but carries far fewer risks.

Ephedrine

Ephedrine, which is similar to the substance amphetamine, which is commonly used in decongestants, has become a popular "herbal" recreational drug. Ephedrine has become a widely marketed performance-enhancing drug. Ephedrine causes all the signs of an overall activation of the secondary nervous system, including an increase in heart rate and blood pressure, dilation of the bronchioles, and an increase in glucose and fatty acids in the circulation. This natural substance is a popular weight loss aid because it causes a breakdown of fat and is thought to suppress appetite. Additionally, some athletes take ephedrine before working out because they believe that it will provide them with greater energy, build lean muscle, enhance their metabolism, and help them burn fat. Some athletes believe that using ephedrine will increase their workout intensity. These beliefs are not substantiated, and there is no evidence that ephedrine actually enhances athletic performance.

Ephedrine has been reported to cause physical and psychological dependence when taken over long periods of time. Additionally, ephedrine can be extremely dangerous and have serious health consequences, especially when combined with caffeine or exercise. Ephedrine used during exercise creates a risk for overstimulating the heart, which can be fatal. Side effects have included chest pain, heart attacks, strokes, seizures, heat stroke, and even death. In response to these risks, the NCAA banned the use of ephedrine in 1997. The FDA finally recognized the dangers of ephedrine and banned the substance in 2004 because of the growing number of fatalities.

Energy Foods

While student-athletes can get the required nutrients and fuel that their body needs through a well-balanced diet, many student-athletes choose to supplement their diet and boost their performance by consuming energy foods and drinks such as energy bars, sports drinks, or gel packs. The past two decades have seen a boom in the use of energy foods in the world of competitive sports. Energy foods come in various shapes, sizes, flavors, and textures. They include candy bars fortified with caffeine, vitamins, and minerals, such as the Snickers Charged and Snickers Marathon Energy Bars, energy bars that are packed with protein, like Clif Bars or PowerBars, and drinks that are enhanced with sodium and potassium, such as Gatorade, and these are just a few. Energy fuels can actually act as an ergogenic aid for athletes, helping to enhance their performance. For example, many student-athletes drink sports drinks during intense exercise, especially when they sweat a lot, because these drinks will quickly replace the electrolytes in their bodies. Distance runners or cyclists may consume gel packs or energy bars during races to replenish carbohydrates and give them extra fuel to compete for a longer duration. Energy foods are also used by some athletes directly after competition to help them replenish the fuel that they used during their workout and to aid in muscle recovery.

There are several advantages to using energy bars for performance enhancement. They are convenient and readily available in groceries, drug stores, training facilities, and even campus bookstores. They have a long shelf life and can be easily carried along to away games or meets. In a pinch, these bars can serve as a mini-meal replacement because of their well-rounded nutrient composition.

Energy drinks, commonly sold in health and nutrition stores, are usually anything but healthful. These drinks contain a variety of ingredients such as caffeine, guarana, taurine, vitamins, a range of amino acids, and many other components that claim to give the consumer a great deal of energy and increase metabolism. The claims and marketing strategies vary, but the dangers are similar. Energy drinks are not regulated by the Food and Drug Administration, so there is really no way of knowing everything that they contain, even if you read the label. The extreme levels of stimulants, vitamins, herbs, and amino acids can be unhealthy and cause serious and unintended side effects. While most of the drinks cause the intended effects, increased energy and alertness, the effect on each person is different. Negative side effects such as gastrointestinal irritation, increased heart rate, anxiety, tremors, and loss of sleep continue to be drawbacks to these energy drinks. Additionally, caffeine is on the banned substance list, and with caffeinated energy drinks, the threshold for a positive test can easily be surpassed.

While there are many positives to supplementing your diet with energy foods and drinks, as with any ergogenic aid, you should evaluate them critically, weighing both the pros and cons before deciding whether or not to use them. As a student-athlete it is important that you understand what exactly is in the energy product. You should read and understand the nutritional label. For example, some of the energy bars are high in sugar, which could give you a quick burst of energy but cause you to crash quickly after eating it. Other energy bars have a high fat content, and there may be better food choices that will meet your needs. Also, you may discover that you get the same results from eating regular, unprocessed foods such as fresh fruit or peanut butter, and you may have an easier time digesting these foods than processed energy bars. One other drawback to using energy foods to supplement your diet is the cost associated with them. The energy foods industry is huge, and billions of dollars are spent each year by consumers looking to find the perfect energy food that will boost their performance and give them a competitive edge.

Human Growth Hormone

One of the most important hormones in the human body is the human growth hormone (HGH). This hormone is made in the pituitary gland, a pea-sized gland that sits in a protected pocket in the center of the brain. It travels through the body and is involved with a variety of body processes pertaining to strength and growth, bone strength, tissue repair, and protein formation, all obviously areas of interest to athletes.

While HGH is produced naturally within the body, it can also be injected. There are documented benefits of HGH. It is effective at making people bigger and stronger and enables people to break down body fat and use it as energy; however, the risks far outweigh the benefits. First, HGH is very costly. Injections must be taken over time to be effective, and a one-month supply can approach $5,000. Also, several serious health consequences are associated with injecting additional HGH into the body. The most disastrous side effect of using HGH is the disease acromegaly, which is a disease of excessive growth and disfigurement. Acromegaly causes the hands and feet to enlarge and the jaw and forehead to protrude. In addition, the use of HGH can cause heart and metabolic problems as well.

THINK ABOUT IT ✔

- ❏ Despite the negative side effects, why might an athlete feel pressured to use an ergogenic aid?

- ❏ Considering each of the eight common ergogenic aids discussed what long-term consequences or stresses both physiologically and psychologically may result from use?

- ❏ What is your view on the use of ergogenic aids in sports? For instance, if your teammates and/or opponents were using them, do you see this as cheating? Why or why not?

The use of HGH is banned by the NCAA as well as other athletic governing bodies; however, it is difficult to detect if an athlete is injecting the hormone. Because the hormone is found naturally in the body, there is currently no test to detect if athletes are using supplements of the hormone. As a student-athlete, you need to be educated about the risks of using HGH because the consequences are serious and in most cases outweigh the performance and physical benefits associated with elevated amounts of HGH in the bloodstream.

Student-Athletes and Ergogenic Aids

Regulation and Safety Issues

Federal laws require manufacturers of dietary supplements to ensure that the products on the market are safe; however, manufacturers are not required to have their supplements and products reviewed by the Food and Drug Administration (FDA) prior to their release. Under the Dietary Supplement Health and Education Act, the FDA can review the product only after it is released. The FDA must show that the product is unsafe before it can take action to restrict the product's use. With the growing number of supplements on the market and fewer regulatory restrictions, there is potential for quality control problems in this industry. For example, the FDA has identified several manufacturers who were using ingredients without testing them to determine their safety. While the FDA is trying to regulate the information that is provided to the consumer after the supplements have reached the market, there is still no guarantee that products are safe and effective.

The FDA does not strictly regulate the supplement industry; therefore, the purity and long-term safety of supplements, such as creatine or amino acid complexes, are unknown. Thus, consumers need to be extremely cautious regarding their use of supplements. Student-athletes in particular must be careful because the NCAA has banned many of the ingredients in these supplements. The NCAA is the strictest governing agency in the athletic community. It conducts thorough and random drug tests checking for a laundry list of banned drugs.

Rules That Govern Ergogenic Aid Usage

The NCAA views participation in sports as a privilege, not a right; therefore, all participants in Division I NCAA sports and Division II schools with postseason competition must agree to be tested on a year-round basis. The urine test screens for anabolic agents, diuretics, ephedrine, peptide hormones, and urine manipulators or masking agents. NCAA tests are conducted by the National Center for Drug Free Sport, which is required to give no more than forty-eight hours' notice to the institution and athletes who have been randomly selected to be tested. In the past, drug testing began in August and ran through the end of the academic year. Due to a change in NCAA legislation, as of June 2006, new drug testing policies were adopted and any student-athlete can be randomly selected to be drug tested at any point throughout the year, including the summer months. Additionally, random testing traditionally occurs during NCAA championship events for participants. It is possible for a student-athlete to be tested more than once a year on campus and at an NCAA championship event.

The privilege of playing a collegiate sport can be revoked at any time for reasons ranging from academic issues to violations of professional/amateur status, but a positive drug test carries the strictest consequences. Student-athletes caught using banned substances are suspended from regular-season and postseason competition for one calendar year. The student-athletes are also charged with the loss of at least one season of competition in all sports. A second positive test renders them ineligible for any remaining seasons of eligibility in all sports. The NCAA is vigilant about drug testing, which helps to create a safer environment for student-athletes. As a result of their strict policies on banned substances, less than 1 percent of student-athletes are found to use drugs. The testing is too rigorous and random, and the consequences too dire for most student-athletes to take the risk.

The NCAA does not have any tolerance for ignorance when student-athletes claim to not be aware of using banned substances. However, many nutritional supplements contain banned substances; thus a student-athlete could unwittingly fail a drug test and automatically be ineligible. Any time a student-athlete uses any type of supplement it is at his or her own risk; therefore, student-athletes should ask and consult with their institution's team physician or athletic trainer before trying any such substance.

In addition to the NCAA, colleges and universities also may have random drug testing for student-athletes. The penalties that come along with a positive test administered at an institution have consequences that differ from the penalties incurred by testing positive on an NCAA test. Each school's policy is different, but penalties for offenses can range from consequences such as notification of guardians and entering a treatment or counseling program to more severe punishments such as suspension or dismissal from the team. Another way institutional tests differ from those administered by the NCAA is that each university or college can test for a different selection of banned substances. For example, not all NCAA tests include marijuana in their screen, since it is not a performance-enhancing drug. But most institutionally administered tests do look for street drugs such as marijuana because they are illegal and detrimental to the health of student-athletes. Knowing this, it is important to remember that student-athletes are subject to random selection for intuitional tests at any point during the year in addition to NCAA tests.

As you well know, concerns exist about banned substances across the athletic spectrum. All major sports and athletic associations have banned substance regulations. You can find them in professional organizations including the International Olympic Movement, World Anti-Doping Agency, U.S. Olympics, United States Anti-Doping Agency, and so on. The major sports orga-

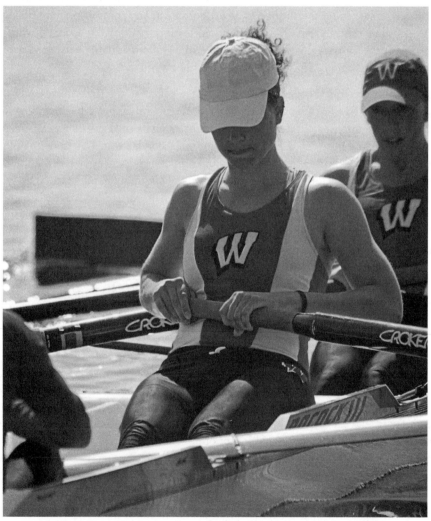

© Geoffrey Kuchera/ShutterStock, Inc.

nizations have regulatory bodies such as the Major Baseball League Players Association, the National Football League Players Association, and World Wrestling Entertainment. Finally, organizations dedicated to high school athletics have regulatory bodies: the National Interscholastic Athletic Administrators Association and the National Federation of High Schools. The book's web site lists Internet resources as well as links to twenty-two sports organizations that address concerns related to ergogenic aids.

Knowing the Facts About Ergogenic Aids

When deciding to use an ergogenic aid, a student-athlete must ask three questions. Is it effective? Is it safe? Is it legal? If the answer is "no" to any one of those questions, it makes sense that it is a good idea to avoid the substance or aid. Unfortunately, some athletes decide to use unsafe or banned substances despite the consequences. These athletes understand that it is not legal, but they believe they can get away with using it. The truth is that tests for banned substances are very effective. If a student-athlete uses a commercial "screen" or masking agents to try to beat a drug test, chances are he or she will still be caught.

As specimen collection procedures and lab analysis technologies improve, an even greater percentage will be caught trying to cheat or beat the test. Cheaters will ultimately be caught during the urine collection process or when the lab results come back. Even with current advanced testing procedures, some student-athletes attempt to use masking agents to pass their drug tests. Masking agents do little more than dilute a urine sample. For instance, some students will drink vinegar in an attempt to lower the pH of urine. What they don't realize is that this procedure will give the lab evidence of tampering. Students who would actually drink enough vinegar to sufficiently "mask" a sample would experience violent diarrhea. Another common misconception is that taking large doses of vitamin C will create a false negative result for marijuana, amphetamines, and barbiturates. Unfortunately, ingesting larges does of vitamin C could actually interact with these drugs and increase the likelihood of a positive test. Additionally, student-athletes may also believe these myths:

- Eating red meat will raise creatine levels in a diluted sample.

- Dog urine can be substituted to pass a drug test.

- Increasing your metabolism will reduce the amount of time a drug can be detected in your system, and eating a high-calorie diet and starting an intense exercise program will do the same.

Making good decisions regarding the use of ergogenic aids and supplements requires educating oneself about the costs, benefits, and risks. Below are five myths about ergogenic aids to help you increase your knowledge on this topic and help you make healthy decisions regarding the use of ergogenic aids.

- *Myth 1:* Special supplements improve athletic performance.

  Fact: Athletes often believe that "ergogenic aids" such as bee pollen, ginseng, brewer's yeast, and DNA will give them a competitive edge. Most of these supplements are expensive, bear no evidence that they improve performance, and may even be harmful to both health and performance.

- *Myth 2:* Consuming large amounts of protein or protein supplements will increase muscle size and strength.

  Fact: Excess protein will not increase muscle growth or strength. When excess protein is consumed, it is either burned as energy or converted to fat.

- *Myth 3:* Amino acid supplements increase muscle mass and decrease body fat.

  Fact: Eating a variety of high-quality protein foods provides most athletes with far more amino acids than they can obtain through supplements.

- *Myth 4:* Protein is for weightlifters.

  Fact: High-protein meals eaten on the day of the event contribute little to energy production and performance. High-protein foods stay in the stomach a long time and can cause indigestion, nausea, and even vomiting if eaten within a few hours of competition.

- *Myth 5:* Steroids are a good way to build muscle.

  Fact: Steroids can stunt an athlete's growth, deepen the voice, cause acne, alter the sex organs, and cause liver damage. The use of steroids is illegal in athletic competitions.

Benefits, Consequences, and Ethics

Student-athletes should feel privileged to participate in athletics because many students strive to compete at the collegiate level, but only a few make the team. Thus, student-athletes are held to very high standards, fall under many pressures, and have tremendous performance demands. Many student-athletes would do anything to enhance their performance and gain an advantage over their opponents; as a result, more student-athletes use ergogenic aids.

Obviously, there are advantages to using some ergogenic aids such as caffeine, dietary supplements, and creatine. Athletes may find themselves getting stronger and faster or having longer endurance, but with these performance gains comes a price. Athletes who use ergogenic aids are subject to scrutiny as there is controversy around whether or not ergogenic aids give student-athletes an unfair advantage. For instance, some players argue that there is free interplay between competitive athletes, and athletes should be able to use training tools and supplements to achieve their performance goals. But, others argue that any type of ergogenic aid can create an unfair playing field. A final argument is that ergogenic aids are fair but only if everyone has equal access to them. These arguments raise an ethical dilemma and elicit the question, should athletes who have used any type of ergogenic aid be allowed to compete with life-long drug-free athletes?

Several years ago the fame of baseball legend Mark McGwire addressed this very question. Mark McGwire was renowned for chasing the Major League Baseball home run record. With his success and recognition, he received a lot of scrutiny. During his career, McGwire used androstenedione, a substance banned by the NCAA but not by Major League Baseball. While technically "legal" in baseball, androstenedione is a steroid predecessor and the ethics of its use as a natural supplement are debatable. McGwire's success has fueled an ethical debate surrounding ergogenics and sports performance supplements. To this day, people argue whether or not McGwire's record is accurate and ethical. Many athletes feel that because McGwire did not break any laws, his accomplishments were fair. Consequently, it is not publicly known if other baseball players took androstenedione. Furthermore, most coaches, teammates, and fans lose respect for athletes who use steroids on any level. They believe that performance-enhancing substances taint the game and lead to unfair competition.

Similar situations cause us to examine issues of legality and morality. For example, it is unfortunate that some athletes who train for lengthy periods of time in the weight room do not always see the same positive gains as teammates or opponents who use ergogenic aids. Many student-athletes grapple with the dilemma of whether or not they should try ergogenic aids and to what extent. Those who use supplements find it is easy to become dependent on them. After all, usage can enhance their performance; however, users must examine their level of ergogenic aids usage as it may become either physically or ethically detrimental to their career. Therefore, if you know a teammate is using supplements, it is important to be open-minded and listen to their reasons for usage. After hearing your teammate's opinion, it is important to share yours, even if you consider supplement usage to be cheating because it creates an unfair advantage. Next, ask your teammate questions about how much they really know about the supplement they are taking and whether or not it is banned by the NCAA. Then suggest that your teammate consult the team athletic trainer or a sports nutritionist. Finally, you can encourage your teammate to review their commitment to the university code of ethics in regard to usage of supplements, and if your university does not have a policy, encourage them to adopt their own personal code of ethics.

Sociocultural factors play a role in supplement usage. To understand why people use supplements and aids, it is important to break down the common misperceptions and incorrect information that athletes use for justification. For instance, your college teammate may have belonged to a high school team where the team collectively agreed on the positive effects of certain supplements. Now, at the college level, it may be difficult for this athlete to discontinue using this substance for fear that it will limit his or her performance. Additionally, you may face a situation where teammates are trying to convince you to try an ergogenic aid. You must make a decision to not give in to them. Instead, you must learn the facts about the social and physical consequences of supplement usage and educate them. You can obtain this information from your coach, athletic department, or university health center.

THINK ABOUT IT

- ❏ Talk with your teammates about their opinions and stance on the NCAA policy regarding random testing of college athletes. Do you think random drug testing causes stress for both athletes and coaches?

- ❏ Do you feel using legal NCAA-regulated supplements to enhance performance and shorten workouts is an effective use of time management?

- ❏ What would you do if you caught a teammate using illegal NCAA-regulated substances?

PLUGGED IN TO SPORTS

Student-Athletes and Technology

Ergogenic aids are defined as any substance, food, chemical, or training method that helps the body work harder and perform better. Mechanical ergogenic aids include devices, apparel, and training equipment. They range from titanium golf clubs, to cork bats, to ultra-light racing flats, to sleeping chambers that simulate high-altitude training. Many athletes seek the latest gadgets, equipment, and gizmos to give them that competitive edge. Whether it be a GPS (global positioning system) watch that a distance runner uses to map his course and track his miles, or a heart rate monitor that a swimmer uses to make sure she trains with enough aerobic intensity, or a weight belt that helps you squat more in the weight room without hurting your back, technology is part of your workout. Researchers continually try to improve fabrics, use the latest materials, and develop new ways to track and monitor performance.

Technology can enhance how you practice and train, having an ergogenic effect. But, like other ergogenic aids, there is some ethical debate around using mechanical, technology-driven aids. Not everyone has the same access to technology and not everyone can afford the latest training devices. Think about some of the equipment you have as a collegiate athlete. Were these same resources available to you as a high school athlete? Do people at other schools have access to these same training tools?

Chapter Summary

Ergogenic aids are substances, techniques, or devices designed to enhance your work output or performance. Ergogenic aids can be mechanical, psychological, pharmacological, physiological, or nutritional. Mechanical aids include apparel and high-tech equipment that give us an advantage. Psychological aids include prayer, meditation, and rituals that athletes do to prepare mentally or spiritually for competition. Pharmacological aids are drugs and synthetic substances, such as steroids, that allow athletes to increase their strength, speed, or ability. Physiological aids, such as blood doping or altitude training, actually allow athletes to alter the way their body functions, allowing them to increase their work capacity, endurance, or performance. Finally, nutritional aids include items that athletes eat, such as energy bars or water with vitamin supplements, that help them fuel their bodies for exercise and recovery.

The term *ergogenic aid* covers a variety of different products, techniques, and substances, and range from caffeine to steroids. They can be safe or unsafe, legal or illegal. Some are readily available and inexpensive while others are harder to obtain, illegal, or very costly. People have different views or beliefs regarding the use of supplements, performance enhancers, and ergogenic aids in sports. Ultimately, it is up to each individual student-athlete to decide what he or she is willing to use. As a student-athlete, you are under a lot of pressure to perform at a collegiate level. Along the way, you will probably wish to try different types of ergogenic aids to enhance your performance. Ultimately, it is your decision whether or not to use an ergogenic aid. Your decision is critical because while some ergogenic aids are safe and welcomed by athletic trainers and coaches, others are banned by the NCAA and can be extremely harmful. Use of these aids could cost you your season, your scholarship, and possibly your career.

When deciding whether or not to use an ergogenic aid, you must ask yourself three questions: Is the substance or technique effective? Is it safe? And is it legal? If you hesitate when answering these questions, or answer "no" to any of these questions, you should not use the ergogenic aid. You need to consider the moral, physical, and psychological consequences of your decisions.

Your Thoughts

1. It can be difficult to tell when companies make false claims about their products' ergogenic properties. Identify some false claims made by ergogenic aid manufacturers. Have your teammates ever told you a false claim about something they were taking? What makes these claims too good to be true? How can you find out more about a product's claims before taking a supplement?

2. Do you believe that ergogenic aids help athletes enhance the ability they already have, or do they provide athletes with artificial gains that could not be achieved otherwise? Discuss your views on artificial gains.

3. Many student-athletes report first hearing about steroids when they were in elementary and middle school. Some report feeling pressure to use steroids. What is the best way for young athletes as well as college students to resist the pressure to enhance their performance by using steroids?

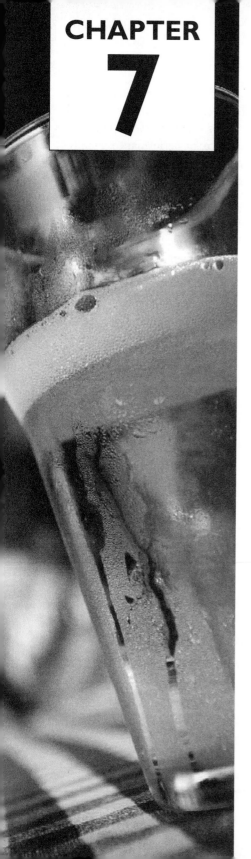

CHAPTER 7

Challenge #5: Alcohol

Learning Objectives

After completing this chapter, you will be able to:

- *Understand the physical effects of alcohol on the body and on athletic performance*

- *Understand and calculate blood alcohol content (BAC)*

- *Identify signs of problem drinking and risky drinking behavior*

- *Locate resources available to help people who are struggling with alcohol abuse and identify warning signs that someone may need help*

© Photos.com

Student-Athletes Say:

- I think parties at college are pathetic. People get high or drunk, act like idiots, hurt people's feelings, and then start the whole cycle over again the next day.

- While I was at a party, someone slipped something into my drink. I passed out from the drug. I do not remember anything but waking up in my friend's dorm room. I felt horrible. She told me she had never seen me so out of control. God only knows what would have happened if she hadn't taken me home.

- Freshman year, I became really good friends with the girl next door. I started to have feelings for her, but I was too nervous to tell her. One night, we ended up at the same party. After a couple drinks, I finally had the courage to tell her how I felt.

- Homecoming weekend is the best weekend on campus. Everyone comes out to tailgate before the football game, and it feels like the whole campus supports our team. After the game, the whole team celebrates. We party and drink all night.

- I never realized before I came to college how many people drink and drive. I see people leaving bars and getting behind the wheel all the time. How could people be so stupid? Don't they realize they could kill themselves or someone else?

- My roommate and I got off to a bad start. My first weekend on campus, I had a volleyball tournament early Saturday morning. I stayed in Friday night to make sure I got a good night's rest. Unfortunately, my plan was ruined when my roommate came stumbling home at 2:00 a.m., woke me up, and got sick in our room. I was so angry that we didn't talk for a week.

Alcohol use is an issue on college campuses throughout the country. Many college students drink. They spend lots of money on alcohol. In addition to the peer pressure to drink alcohol on campus, students are constantly reminded through advertisements in the media that life goes better with a drink. With a drink you can be anyone you want: successful, pretty, handsome, desirable, sexy, outgoing, and rich. From the advertisements, it seems you would need to be crazy not to drink at least occasionally, if not often.

The concern for student-athletes is that they often find themselves in an environment with easy access to alcohol and with people who are drinking. The perception is that drinking is fun. Drinking can feel relaxing and for some, it is a way to be social with friends as well as a way to meet new people and make new friends. And although you might have drank in high school, being on a college campus away from parents and family with newfound freedom and fewer restrictions presents challenges for even the most disciplined and aware person. Plus, even if you are under the legal drinking age of twenty-one, drinking might be legal for older teammates and classmates. And finally, even if you are not drinking, you can be affected by the drinking behavior of others in the form of accidents, poor performance, and unwanted sexual advances.

This chapter focuses on the decisions you are already making about the role of alcohol in your life. As you complete the Student-Athlete Challenge #5: Alcohol Self-Assessment in Box 7.1, consider the availability and access to alcohol on your campus (even if you are underaged). Are you faced every day with invitations to hang out and party where there is alcohol? As a student-athlete are you concerned about alcohol? What do your coaches and teammates say about drinking alcohol?

Box 7.1. Student-Athlete Challenge #5: *Alcohol Self-Assessment*

Directions: Evaluate each statement on a scale of 1 to 5, from 1 being "never" to 5 being "almost always." For each statement evaluate if your behavior adds value (+), is neutral (0), or decreases value (−) in regard to your student-athlete success in regard to your classes and sport.

Statement	Never			Almost Always		Value Added		
	1	2	3	4	5	+	0	−
1. I get into fights or arguments when I drink.	☐	☐	☐	☐	☐	☐	☐	☐
2. I do things when I drink that I later regret.	☐	☐	☐	☐	☐	☐	☐	☐
3. Family and friends question me about how often and how much I drink.	☐	☐	☐	☐	☐	☐	☐	☐
4. I black out and/or vomit when I drink.	☐	☐	☐	☐	☐	☐	☐	☐
5. I get behind the wheel of a car after having a few drinks.	☐	☐	☐	☐	☐	☐	☐	☐
6. When my friends and I hang out together, there is alcohol involved.	☐	☐	☐	☐	☐	☐	☐	☐
7. When I drink, I play drinking games.	☐	☐	☐	☐	☐	☐	☐	☐
8. Upperclassmen supply underage people on our team with alcohol.	☐	☐	☐	☐	☐	☐	☐	☐
9. I feel that drinking alcohol has a negative impact on my ability to reach my goals.	☐	☐	☐	☐	☐	☐	☐	☐
10. Although my team has a drinking rule/policy during the season, people break the rules.	☐	☐	☐	☐	☐	☐	☐	☐
11. I feel pressure to drink.	☐	☐	☐	☐	☐	☐	☐	☐
12. When I drink, I drink to get drunk.	☐	☐	☐	☐	☐	☐	☐	☐

Drinking alcohol is something you may have seen and experienced growing up. Whether or not drinking alcohol was part of your family experience, or is part of your life now, drinking alcohol is part of our culture. Family celebrations, watching sports, after work or school, and hanging out with friends are all occasions when some enjoy having a glass of wine, a can of beer, a shot, or a mixed drink.

> *I was nervous about the start of soccer season. I played for the same coach for the past four years and I was best friends with all the girls on my high school team. I knew there would be a lot of new things to get adjusted to as I joined my new team. I wanted more than anything to make the starting lineup and win the respect of my new teammates. The first game of the season, I was performing at my peak. Not only was I the only freshman starting player, but I scored the game's winning goal. I was so excited. I knew I had managed to impress my teammates. After the game, in the locker room, the captain and some of the other star players asked me to go with them to a party. When I arrived, everyone was drinking. I knew we had an early practice the next day and I probably should not drink, but how was I supposed to say no to the captain? She handed me a shot of alcohol and she wanted to toast our team's victory. I hesitated for a minute, but I did not want to be the only one not drinking. I figured, how could I get in trouble when the rest of the starters were drinking too? If coach found out, he would not bench the entire starting lineup. I ended up drinking with the other girls all night. Unfortunately, my body did not handle the alcohol that well because the next day I performed horribly at practice and felt miserable. My coach told me if I continued to perform poorly, I would not be able to have a lot of playing time on the field.*

As a college student-athlete you are part of the most easily identifiable group of individuals by faculty, students, parents, community members, administration, college trustees, alumni, and media. You are known by people you have never met. This chapter is based in the reality that your decisions about the use of alcohol can become public quickly. And whether or not you drink, others around you are drinking. The chapter is focused on getting you the information and support you need to make the choices you want about the role of alcohol in your life.

Understanding Alcohol Consumption

The most widely used drug on college campuses is alcohol. Surveys show that 81 percent of college students use or have used alcohol, and 44 percent of these students have engaged in risky drinking (consuming at least five drinks in a single sitting). Alcohol is heavily used by many college students because it is readily available and often socially encouraged. Many students drink because they perceive that everyone else is doing it and that it is a fun, unavoidable aspect of college culture. Drinking alcohol, students expect a good time. Some students drink because they are trying to fit in or because they feel pressure to drink in order to fit into a social

THINK ABOUT IT ✔

❑ Do you think drinking is a problem on your campus? Why do you think so many college students participate in underage drinking?

❑ Think about a friend, classmate, or teammate who drinks a lot. Does it seem that drinking has a negative impact on their ability to reach their goals?

group. Finally, some students use alcohol as a way to cope with the stresses and pressures they encounter in college. Faced with a busy schedule, demanding classes, practices, games, and expectations from parents, professors, and coaches, some student-athletes adopt a "work hard, play hard" mentality and attempt to unwind and relieve their stress through alcohol. No matter what the underlying issue is for alcohol consumption, it is a growing problem on college campuses as incidences of high-risk drinking (consuming at least five drinks in a single sitting) and alcohol-related accidents and problems are on the rise.

The Effects of Alcohol

An Introduction to Alcohol

Because alcohol is legal for some students and accessible, many perceive it to be harmless; however, this is not the case. Contrary to popular opinion, alcohol use can have serious consequences. Impairment begins with the first drink, and you may be surprised to learn that 12 ounces of beer, 5 ounces of wine, or 1 1/2 ounces of liquor constitutes "one drink." Therefore, even moderate drinking, having even a single can of beer, affects performance. For example, people who consume alcohol experience impaired motor coordination for 12 to 18 hours after use and decreased aerobic capacity for 48 hours. Alcohol also impacts a person's fuel and energy levels. Alcohol is a poor nutritional source of carbohydrates for the body. In fact, rather than fueling your body, alcohol dehydrates you and impairs fluid levels. In addition, the body metabolizes alcohol in the liver. This disrupts the regular function of the liver, producing glycogen. Glycogen is a basic fuel for the body, so when production is interrupted, the body is faced with less fuel and becomes fatigued. The breaking down of alcohol in the body is a slow process. Alcohol is metabolized in the liver at a rate of only 10 to 15 milliliters or 0.5 ounces per hour. Therefore, the more you drink, the more intoxicated you become, the longer alcohol remains in your body, and the longer you will experience the effects. The only thing that can sober you up is time.

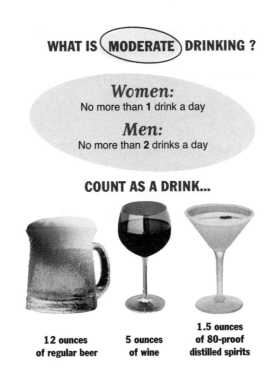

WHAT IS (MODERATE) DRINKING ?

Women:
No more than **1** drink a day

Men:
No more than **2** drinks a day

COUNT AS A DRINK...

**12 ounces
of regular beer**

**5 ounces
of wine**

**1.5 ounces
of 80-proof
distilled spirits**

Figure 7.1
Source: Courtesy of USDA Center for Nutrition Policy and Promotion

The amount of alcohol in a drink can be hard to determine. For example, a mixed drink and beer may both be served in pint glasses; however, depending on how strong the mixed drink is made, the mixed drink may contain up to three times the amount of alcohol as a pint of beer. Figure 7.1 illustrates what "one drink" is equal to:

- 12 ounces of beer

- 1.5 ounces of liquor

- 5 ounces of wine

Unfortunately, many college students are misinformed when it comes to the effects, consequences, and realities of alcohol use. In Box 7.2 is a list of common statements about alcohol. The correct answers are listed. Can you explain why the statements are true or false?

Does your team have a drinking rule or policy about alcohol during the season? Many coaches make strict rules regarding alcohol use during the season, not to spoil your fun or

STUDENT REFLECTION

STUDENT REFLECTION

Box 7.2. Do you know why these are true or false?

1. Alcohol enters the bloodstream primarily through the stomach.	False
2. Alcohol chills the body.	True
3. A mixed drink with one shot (1.5 ounces) of liquor has more alcohol than a 5-ounce glass of wine.	False
4. Mixing alcohol with over-the-counter drugs such as cold medicine or acetaminophen can be dangerous.	True
5. Mixing alcohol with carbonated beverages such as soda makes you feel the effects of alcohol faster.	True
6. I can drink and still be in control.	False
7. The liver metabolizes alcohol at a constant rate of one standard drink per hour.	True
8. Blacking out causes people to forget what happened while they were drinking.	True
9. Blood alcohol content is affected by body size, the amount of alcohol consumed, and the rate of drinking.	True
10. The physiological effects of alcohol last up to 48 hours.	True

dictate your choices but to look out for your safety as well as your ability to compete to the best of your ability. When student-athletes drink alcohol, it depletes their bodies' vital fuel and leads to the early onset of muscle fatigue during games or workouts. Also, without enough glycogen, muscle tissue does not have the energy to repair its cells after strenuous exercise. Because the effects of alcohol last up to 48 hours, it is important to pay close attention to when you consume any form of alcohol. You may think it is fine to drink a day or two before a big competition, but your body can still be negatively affected. For example, a football player who drinks moderately on a Thursday night may still experience the side effects of alcohol during his game on Saturday. Alcohol robs the brain of its food, glucose. The football player may experience impaired reaction time and hand–eye coordination. This is certainly not going to help him read the quarterback's throw or make a hard catch. Perception is distorted, which affects an athlete's accuracy. For example, our football player may have a hard time with precise footwork and running complicated play patterns.

Athletes also experience a decrease in strength and aerobic capacity when they consume alcohol. In the case of the football player mentioned previously, he will not only have difficulty catching the ball, but also have difficulty mustering up the energy to speed down the field, outrun his defender, and make it into the end zone. In addition to hindering athletic skill and performance, alcohol also affects an athlete's ability to regulate body temperature. This poses a real threat when athletes compete in extreme temperatures. For example, if our football player is competing on a very cold day, he may become severely dehydrated because his body isn't prepared to regulate temperature and fluid effectively.

Knowing Your Limits

Set foot on any college campus and you will probably hear at least one student say, "I've only had a few drinks, I'm still okay to drive," or "Drinking six drinks in an evening doesn't mean I'm a binge drinker, it just means that I have a really high tolerance for alcohol." For some reason, many college students feel that they are immune to the effects of alcohol consumption, when in fact, alcohol has definite physiological effects on the body.

The effects of alcohol are measured by a person's blood alcohol content (BAC) or blood alcohol concentration, the concentration of alcohol in blood. It is measured as a percentage by mass, by mass per volume, or a combination. For example, a BAC of 0.02 percent can mean 2 grams of alcohol per 1,000 grams of an individual's blood, or it can mean 0.2 grams of alcohol per 100 milliliters of blood. The number of drinks consumed is a very poor measure of intoxication largely because of variation in physiology and individual alcohol tolerance. However, it is generally accepted that the consumption of two standard drinks (containing a total of 20 grams) of alcohol will increase the average person's BAC roughly 0.05 percent (a single standard drink consumed each hour after the first two will keep the BAC at approximately 0.05 percent), but there is much variation according to body weight, gender, and body fat percentage. Furthermore, tolerance to alcohol varies from one person to another and can be affected by such factors as genetics, adaptation to chronic alcohol use, and synergistic effects of drugs.

Figure 7.2 outlines the effects that alcohol has on the body as BAC increases. Notice that there are separate charts for females and males. It is generally accepted that your body's BAC depends on four key factors:

- Your sex

- Your weight

- Number of drinks

- Rate of consumption

Men
BODY WEIGHT IN POUNDS

DRINKS	100	120	140	160	180	200	220	240	
			APPROXIMATE BLOOD ALCOHOL PERCENTAGE						
0	.00	.00	.00	.00	.00	.00	.00	.00	ONLY SAFE DRIVING LIMIT
1	.04	.03	.03	.02	.02	.02	.02	.02	IMPAIRMENT BEGINS
2	.08	.06	.05	.05	.04	.04	.03	.03	DRIVING SKILLS AFFECTED
3	.11	.09	.08	.07	.06	.06	.05	.05	
4	.15	.12	.11	.09	.08	.08	.07	.06	POSSIBLE CRIMINAL PENALTIES
5	.19	.16	.13	.12	.11	.09	.09	.08	
6	.23	.19	.16	.14	.13	.11	.10	.09	
7	.26	.22	.19	.16	.15	.13	.12	.11	LEGALLY INTOXICATED
8	.30	.25	.21	.19	.17	.15	.14	.13	
9	.34	.28	.24	.21	.19	.17	.15	.14	CRIMINAL PENALTIES
10	.38	.31	.27	.23	.21	.19	.17	.16	

Women
BODY WEIGHT IN POUNDS

DRINKS	90	100	120	140	160	180	200	220	240	
				APPROXIMATE BLOOD ALCOHOL PERCENTAGE						
0	.00	.00	.00	.00	.00	.00	.00	.00		ONLY SAFE DRIVING LIMIT
1	.05	.05	.04	.03	.03	.03	.02	.02	.02	IMPAIRMENT BEGINS
2	.10	.09	.08	.07	.06	.05	.05	.04	.04	DRIVING SKILLS AFFECTED
3	.15	.14	.11	.10	.09	.08	.07	.06	.06	
4	.20	.18	.15	.13	.11	.10	.09	.08	.08	POSSIBLE CRIMINAL PENALTIES
5	.25	.23	.19	.16	.14	.13	.11	.10	.09	
6	.30	.27	.23	.19	.17	.15	.14	.12	.11	
7	.35	.32	.27	.23	.20	.18	.16	.14	.13	LEGALLY INTOXICATED
8	.40	.36	.30	.26	.23	.20	.18	.17	.15	
9	.45	.41	.34	.29	.26	.23	.20	.19	.17	CRIMINAL PENALTIES
10	.51	.45	.38	.32	.28	.25	.23	.21	.19	

Note: Subtract 0.01% for each 40 minutes of drinking. Your body can get rid of one drink per hour. One drink is 1.25 oz of 80-proof liquor, 12 oz of beer, or 5 oz of table wine. Data supplied by the Pennsylvania Liquor Control Board.

Figure 7.2
Source: Reproduced from Pennsylvania Liquor Control Board. Used with permission.

Figure 7.3 illustrates the physical impairments associated with an increased BAC. The legal limit for operating a vehicle is a BAC of 0.08 in most states. While penalties vary case by case, a first-time offender of driving under the influence of alcohol (DUI) can face fines up to $500, one year of probation, incarceration for up to six months, license suspension for six months to a year, and car impoundment for ten days. Penalties increase for people who have a BAC over 0.20 or who are second-time offenders.

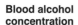

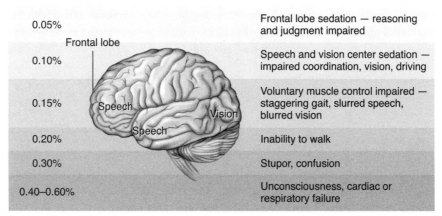

Figure 7.3

Concerns About Drinking

Among student-athletes, alcohol use is a concern. On one hand, the last thing your school, team, coach, and teammates want is for you (or any of your teammates) to have a problem as a result of drinking too much alcohol. On the other hand, addressing a concern is a challenge due to denial, inappropriate behavior, and enabling. Furthermore, it is important for you to know what to do in the event someone consumes too much.

Denial

One of the most difficult challenges in addressing concerns about alcohol among student-athletes (as well as all college students) is denial that alcohol use is a problem. Furthermore,

---

THINK ABOUT IT ✓

- ❑ Using the charts in Figure 7.2, what would the BAC be for a twenty-one-year-old male who weighs 180 pounds and had five drinks in the past two hours? Would he be over the legal limit to drive?

- ❑ Recently, all states have lowered the legal driving BAC from .10 to .08. Do you agree or disagree with this change?

- ❑ Do you think stricter penalties for drunk driving will deter people from drinking and driving? Why or why not?

alcohol use becomes alcohol abuse when it interferes with your school, sport, work, or social and family relationships or when it entails any violation of the law, including driving under the influence. Alcoholism, or alcohol dependency, results when personal and health problems related to alcohol use are severe and stopping alcohol use results in withdrawal symptoms. Some six million Americans can be described as alcoholics.

The tendency of students is to deny that an alcohol problem or abuse exists. Students will rationalize that a couple of drinks are calming or a reward after a hard workout. They intellectualize that they can stop whenever they want. Students use these and any one of a number of strategies to avoid addressing the role of alcohol in their lives and the accompanying anxiety of not having alcohol to help get them through life.

Overcoming denial about an alcohol problem or abuse is thought by many to be the single hardest part of addressing an alcohol concern. Denial acts as a protective shield that gets harder as problems related to drinking increase and people try to help.

Overcoming denial is an internal process that often begins when a person gets scared from hitting a physical, emotional, or mental bottom, develops insight into their problem and tries to correct it, or has an emotional or spiritual awakening that gives them the power to change the way they are living. Overcoming denial often requires help from friends, relatives, or professionals. However, asking for help is one of the hardest actions to take for someone in denial.

Inappropriate Behavior—Drinking Games

A challenge for student-athletes is not to behave inappropriately and in particular to avoid drinking games. Urging others to drink, buying alcohol for others, paying others to buy alcohol for you, or trying to get someone drunk just for the fun of it are all inappropriate behaviors that are dangerous. And while you may think that these behaviors are no big deal, the possible consequences are quite serious and damaging. Drinking games, particularly for student-athletes, can be a problem. In many college environments, drinking is less expensive than most other forms of entertainment. Students say it is cheaper to go to a bar with drink specials than it is to go to a movie. For a few dollars students can drink all night.

Many college students enjoy playing drinking games that encourage excessive alcohol consumption. The games are considered good icebreakers and are sometimes used to reduce social anxiety and get to know people at parties. These games typically involve a set of rules designed to ensure a large consumption of alcohol. Games are now available on the Internet, where Web sites invite users to share their favorites. Playing drinking games increases your rate and volume of consumption and drinking-related problems compared with those of students who do not play the games.

Not participating in inappropriate behavior or playing the games requires you to skillfully resist the pressure to be part of the group and the fun, and you risk ruining the good time. Sometimes it is hard to refuse. You need to think ahead, to plan what you might say and in some cases avoid the situations. You want to be aware of direct pressure to participate in inappropriate behaviors such as being invited to go out drinking. Indirect pressure consists of pressure to be part of the group: glorifying how drunk people are going to get or did get at the last get-together. Finally, you can impose pressure on yourself to be part of the group, accepted and liked by others at the expense of your feelings and own health.

Enabling

Another challenge is not to be an enabler. Enablers want to soften the impact and reduce pain, and as a result, they end up shielding users from the consequences of their drinking. If you are busy cleaning up a teammate's vomit, paying for repairs from damages from an alcohol-fueled fight in your room, or reporting a teammate being sick rather than hung over, you are enabling. Enablers are good people, loyal, loving, and well-intentioned friends and family members. However, their support is misplaced, often motivated by trying to avoid problems and thinking a problem will resolve itself.

The challenge of enabling is that slowly, over time, someone else's drinking problem becomes your problem. Your time and energy are suddenly spent covering up, making excuses, and keeping a secret about someone else's behavior. At first it seems that you are protecting the person, but very quickly, without you necessarily noticing, you are protecting yourself. Not being an enabler requires support. You need to talk with a trusted person (e.g., coach, counselor, professor, teammate, or parent) to figure out how to interpret your behavior while supporting the person to address his or her drinking. It is not your responsibility to solve the person's drinking problem. In reality you cannot. All you can do is set limits about when and how you will support and aid the person. The person needs to be in charge of his or her own life as well as deal with the consequences of drinking.

Alcohol Emergencies

We all know that when people drink too much, they get drunk, and at some point they may even become sick. You may find yourself in difficult situations. Do you know how to help someone who is heavily intoxicated? Many people try to sober up by drinking coffee, taking a cold shower, or getting some fresh air. Unfortunately, these "methods" are ineffective. In reality, the only thing that will sober a person up is time. The body eliminates alcohol at a rate of one drink per hour. Take away your friend's car keys, get the person to a safe place where they cannot harm themselves or others, and give them water to keep their body hydrated. If someone is at the point of becoming ill or passing out, make sure that another person is there to look after them. It is also important to make sure that the person's breathing is not labored or that they are not lying in a position where they could choke or suffocate if they vomited. Finally, recognize when a situation is out of your hands. At that point, it is best to get medical help.

By thinking about consequences of alcohol abuse prior to getting in a critical situation, you will be better able to handle them. Knowing how to handle circumstances such as these may literally mean the difference between life and death. Severe intoxication and/or alcohol poisoning can be quite dangerous. Here are some basic guidelines to help you size up the scene and decide how to help a drunken friend.

DO

- Assist the person to a comfortable and safe place.
- Use a calm, strong voice; be firm.
- Assess if the person is in a life-threatening situation and get help if needed.
- Lay the person down on their side with knees up so they won't choke if they vomit.
- Check breathing every ten minutes. Do not leave the person alone!
- Stay with someone who is vomiting to be sure they don't swallow or breathe in the vomit.

DON'T

- Don't give cold showers.
- Don't try to walk the person around.
- Don't provoke a fight by arguing or laughing at someone who is drunk.
- Don't try to counsel the person—confront the behavior later when they are sober.
- Don't give anything to eat or drink—coffee and food won't help and the person may choke.
- Don't permit the person to drive.
- Don't give any drugs; they will not help sober someone up, and in combination with alcohol they may be lethal.
- Don't induce vomiting.

EMERGENCY GUIDE—Call Safety and Security if:

- The person cannot be aroused by shaking or shouting.
- The person's breathing is shallow, irregular, or slowed to less than 6–7 breaths per minute.

THINK ABOUT IT ✔

❑ Have you ever felt pressured by a friend or teammate to drink excessively? How did you respond to this peer pressure? Would you do anything differently if you were faced with the same situation again?

❑ What are some "hangover cures" student-athletes often try? Knowing the physiological affects of alcohol and the effects that it has on the body, what advice would you give to a student-athlete who has had too much to drink?

❑ How prevalent are drinking games on your campus and within your team? Now that you know the dangers of these games, what are your views on these drinking behaviors? What would you do if your teammates were playing a drinking game and were trying to get you to join in?

- The person drank alcohol in combination with any other drugs.

- The person sustained a blow to the head or any injury that caused bleeding.

- The person drank a large quantity within a short period and then collapsed.

If you are not sure what to do, but think that the person needs help, call for medical advice.

Every school and team needs to determine the threshold of concern with respect to individuals. Or, phrased another way, what the school and team are prepared to overlook. The threshold for concern should be low. Whether an alcohol incident represents an isolated event or a chronic problem will never be outwardly or immediately apparent.

Women and Drinking

Alcoholism, heavy drinking, risky drinking problem drinking, and other drug use were long assumed to be problems of men. Women represent a growing percentage of drinkers, including those with alcohol problems and also those with alcohol dependence. For younger women in the general population, the proportion of drinkers is beginning to equal that of men.

Young women in their twenties and early thirties are more likely to drink than older women. No one factor predicts whether a woman will have problems with alcohol, or at what age she is most at risk. However, some aspects of a woman's life experience seem to make problem drinking more likely. For example, heavy drinking and drinking problems among white women are most common in younger age groups. Among African American women, however, drinking problems are more common in middle age than youth. A woman's ethnic origins—and the extent to which she adopts the attitudes of mainstream versus her native culture—influence how and when she will drink.

THINK ABOUT IT ✔

❑ In your opinion, what is the biggest risk to student-athletes who drink alcohol?

❑ Do you think there are greater risks associated with females who drink alcohol? Why or why not?

For women even moderate drinking can have short- and long-term health effects, both positive and negative:

Benefits

Heart disease: Heart disease, once thought of as a threat mainly to men, is also the leading killer of women in the United States. Drinking moderately may lower risk for coronary heart disease, mainly among women over age 55. However, there are other factors that reduce the risk of heart disease, including maintaining a healthy diet, exercise, not smoking, and keeping a healthy weight. Moderate drinking provides little, if any, net health benefit for younger people. (Heavy drinking can actually damage the heart.)

Risks

Drinking and driving: It doesn't take much alcohol to impair driving ability. The chances of being killed in a single-vehicle crash are increased at a blood alcohol level that a 140-pound woman would reach after having one drink on an empty stomach. The number of female drivers involved in alcohol-related fatal traffic crashes is going up, even as the number of male drivers involved in such crashes has decreased. This trend may reflect the increasing number of women who drive themselves, even after drinking, as opposed to riding as a passenger.

Medication interactions: More than 150 medications interact harmfully with alcohol. For example, any medication that causes drowsiness or sedation—for example, many cough and cold medications—can increase the sedative effects of alcohol. When taking any medication, read package labels and warnings carefully.

Breast cancer: Research suggests that in some women, as little as one drink per day can slightly raise the risk of breast cancer. It's not possible to know how alcohol will affect the risk of breast cancer in any one woman, but with so many new cases of breast cancer each year, even a small increase in risk can have an impact on the number of cases.

Sexual violence and unwanted pregnancy: On college campuses, assaults, unwanted sexual advances, and unplanned and unsafe sex are all more likely among students who drink heavily on occasion—for men five drinks in a row, for women, four.

Among the heaviest drinkers, women equal or surpass men in the number of problems that result from their drinking. For example, female alcoholics have death rates 50–100 percent higher than those of male alcoholics, including deaths from suicides, alcohol-related accidents, heart disease and stroke, and liver cirrhosis.

Gaining Support

Being Media Savvy

You are deluged every day by a steady stream of noise and images. College students are targeted and told what is fun, relevant, and important. High on that list is drinking alcohol. The ads tell us that sports and drinking are made for each other. Many people believe there is a strong relationship between alcohol advertisements and college students' drinking.

On one hand, is there a cause-and-effect relationship between beer commercials and whether people drink or not—whether they're of legal age or underage? Can advertisements really influence people to drink? Frequently you will hear that advertising simply helps those individuals who drink to identify with a brand, and that is why the beer companies advertise. On the other hand, there is no question that the beer producers are competing among each other. However, you do not want to be naive and think that is the only reason for advertising. For example, advertising might also attract new users and encourage current users to increase consumption. What do you think?

Whether fueled by advertising on not, alcohol consumption is a serious problem on college campuses. Who created this message? What creative techniques are used to get your attention? How might different people interpret this message? What lifestyles, values, and points of view are in this message? What was left out and why? Why is this message being sent?

Personal History

A person's genetic makeup shapes how quickly he or she feels the effects of alcohol, how pleasant drinking is for him or her, and how drinking alcohol over the long term will affect health, even the chances that the individual could have problems with alcohol. A family history of alcohol problems, risk of illnesses like heart disease and breast cancer, medications, and age are among the factors for each person to weigh in deciding when, how much, and how often to drink.

When Drinking Becomes a Problem

Drinking alcohol does not come without consequences. And while it may seem fun and harmless, frequently that is not true for many student-athletes. Sometimes it is helpful to think about consequences of drinking. How many times after drinking alcohol during the last year have you experienced any of the problems listed in Box 7.3. What do your answers tell you about

Box 7.3. After drinking alcohol, the number of times you experienced the problem during the last year.

Problem	0	1–2	3–4	5+
1. Had a hangover				
2. Felt nauseated or vomited				
3. Had memory loss				
4. Were injured or hurt				
5. Missed class				
6. Had unprotected sex				
7. Performed poorly on a test or project				
8. Performed poorly in practice				
9. Performed poorly in a competition				
10. Damaged property				
11. Had an argument or fight				
12. Did something you later regretted				
13. Were taken advantage of sexually				
14. Were criticized by someone you know				
15. Were in trouble with police or campus authorities				

your drinking? Talk with your friends and teammates about the consequences of their alcohol consumption.

Some people have not experienced negative consequences from drinking alcohol. However, drinking can still be a problem. A person who may have a drinking problem should answer the following four questions:

- Have you ever felt you should cut down on your drinking?

- Have people annoyed you by criticizing your drinking?

THINK ABOUT IT

- ❑ What are some warning signs that a person may have a drinking problem?

- ❑ Students often receive mixed messages about drinking alcohol. On one hand, there are rules and laws that try to prevent underage students from drinking, but on the other hand, there is advertising for alcohol everywhere we turn. Do you feel that alcohol consumption is tolerated or even encouraged on your campus? What are some ways that your campus sends mixed messages?

- ❑ Where on your campus could students seek help if they identified with the questions above or felt that their use of alcohol has begun negatively impacting their life?

PLUGGED IN TO SPORTS

Student-Athletes and Technology

College students, including student-athletes, are very likely to embrace new technologies, especially when it helps them communicate and socialize with friends. As a result, over two-thirds of college students have a Facebook or MySpace account, and use these sites to chat with friends, post pictures, and stay connected. A favorite feature of these sites is the online photo album. Students upload their photos and share pictures with their friends. They use the site as their personal online photo album. Students literally post hundreds of pictures. Some are as simple as shots from their vacation, some are of friends and families, but a vast majority of the photos are of social events. This may seem harmless. After all, what's wrong with sharing photos among friends? On the surface, there is nothing wrong, but caution should be used. Remember, other people besides your friends can use, access, and even manipulate your photos. In addition, many college students include pictures of partying and even drinking on their sites. It is not uncommon to find references to drinking or underage students holding beer cans or cups in their hands. Whether you are drinking or not in the photo, these photos can be incriminating and inappropriate. As a student-athlete you represent not only yourself but your team and your school. Photos of you online that involve drinking or can even be misconstrued to make it appear that you are participating in irresponsible use of alcohol can have serious ramifications. Some schools have gone so far as to monitor student-athletes' Web pages and have them remove questionable photos. Other schools have banned student-athletes from using these sites at all. The important thing to remember is to not get too caught up in the hype of these sites, protect yourself from letting others exploit you online, and be conscientious about what you post online. As a rule of thumb, don't post something online that you wouldn't want your coach, your mother, or your future employer to see.

- Have you ever felt bad or guilty about your drinking?

- Have you ever had a drink first thing in the morning to steady your nerves or to get rid of a hangover?

One "yes" answer suggests a possible alcohol problem. If you responded "yes" to more than one question, it is very likely that you have a problem with alcohol. In either case, it is important that you see your health care provider right away to discuss your responses to these questions.

Even if you answered "no" to all of the above questions, if you are having drinking-related problems with your classes, practice, performance, relationships, health, or with the law, you should still seek help.

Chapter Summary

Because it is legal and readily available, alcohol has become the most commonly used drug on college campuses. While many students perceive that alcohol consumption is just a normal part of college life, as a student-athlete you need to think twice about your involvement with alcohol. Knowing the effects of alcohol, your personal history, as well as your own limits can keep you in control. This is not always easy in a culture where you are deluged with advertisements telling you that drinking alcohol is fun and cool. According to the ads and promotions, an evening drinking with your friends is less expensive and more fun than any other activity you might think of.

Struggles and problems with alcohol are not always easy to identify. Some student-athletes, maybe you or a friend, say things like, "Everyone drinks," "I can stop any time I want," or "It makes me feel good." These statements may be true or they may be denials that are masking a problem. Likewise, you may be reluctant to address a concern about a friend's or family member's drinking. By avoiding the issue, are you enabling the person's behavior by lying and covering up problems that have resulted from their drinking? Furthermore, female student-athletes need to be especially attentive because of negative consequences related to drinking and driving, sexual violence, and unwanted pregnancies.

Finally, if you think you might have a problem with alcohol or you are concerned about a friend's or family member's drinking, talk to someone you trust. Don't wait to get help. The situation may not get better.

Your Thoughts

1. You have been invited to go out drinking with a group of people you would like to get to know. You like to drink, but they have asked you to be the designated driver. How do you

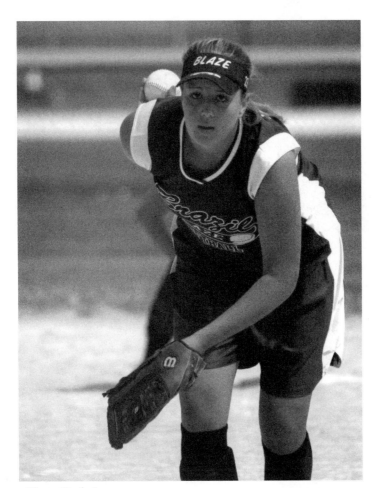

© Lori Carpenter/ShutterStock, Inc.

feel about being the designated driver? Do you think it will be fun? What must these people think of you, if they invited you to be the designated driver?

2. Create or remember a situation when you were at a party and an emergency regarding alcohol arose. What would/did you do? How would/could you handle this situation differently? What are your options? What are some ways you can reduce the harm of drinking and/or doing drugs?

3. For every person who becomes intoxicated, four people are impacted negatively. Give examples of how someone who is drunk can hurt others mentally, physically, or emotionally.

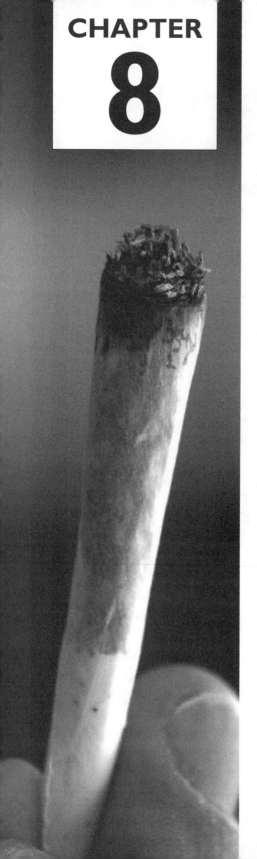

CHAPTER 8

Challenge #6: Tobacco, Marijuana, and Other Drugs

Learning Objectives

After completing this chapter, you will be able to:

- *Understand the physical effects of tobacco, marijuana, and other drugs on the body*

- *Understand how to quit or help someone quit smoking or using tobacco products*

- *Disprove myths about marijuana*

- *Identify and describe the five categories of drugs: depressants, hallucinogens, stimulants, narcotics and inhalants*

© Amihays/ShutterStock, Inc.

Student-Athletes Say:

- I can't imagine going out on the weekends and drinking without having a few cigarettes. It's not like I'm addicted. I just like to smoke socially.

- I did not have a lot of exposure to drugs in high school, and I always assumed that students, especially athletes, didn't use them. During my first week of school, I was shocked when I walked into my dorm room after practice and found my roommate and three of his friends smoking marijuana.

- I was having a hard time sleeping, so a friend gave me pills to help. They worked, but the next day I was drowsy and tired. I had to drink three cups of coffee just to make it though my class. By late afternoon, I needed another boost, so I took a No-Doz pill to stay awake. By the end of the day, I had so many stimulants in my system that it was impossible to fall asleep. Within no time, I had fallen into a cycle of taking sleeping pills at night and uppers all day.

- At finals time I needed a few Adderalls to help me focus. I bought them from a friend in the dorm.

- After my injury I didn't use all the Vicodin the doctors prescribed. Plus they also gave me some Percodan that I also saved and sold. I made some easy money.

- I've smoked pot at parties before. I really don't see what the big deal is; it's not like I'm going to get addicted to it or start using harder drugs.

A s a student-athlete, you live in a world with easy access to a lot of drugs. Today, thousands of drugs are available to you that can be used legally or illegally. Drugs are used for medical reasons, for recreation, and to achieve effects that do not include maintaining health. Student-athletes (same as all college students) sometimes use drugs and may eventually abuse drugs to cope with the pressures of college life. Despite the wealth of knowledge regarding the dangers of unnecessary drug use together with increasing regulations and stiff penalties for violations of the drug laws, many student-athletes use legal and illegal types of drugs without any medically approved reason. Even among student-athletes, who as a group appear dedicated to health and wellness, perceptions and use of drugs vary.

Generally speaking, any substance that modifies the nervous system and state of consciousness is a drug. Such modification enhances, inhibits, or distorts the functioning of the body, thus also affecting the pattern of behavior and social functioning. Psychoactive drugs are classified as either licit (legal) or illicit (illegal). For example, coffee, tea, alcohol, tobacco, and over-the-counter (OTC) drugs are licit. When licit drugs are used in moderation, they often are socially acceptable. Marijuana, cocaine, and LSD are examples of illicit drugs. Any use of these drugs is not generally socially acceptable by the larger society or legally allowed.

This chapter focuses on tobacco and marijuana, the causes of many personal health, social, and economic problems (far more problems than caused by illicit drugs). A chapter section also focuses on the use and abuse by student-athletes of other drugs that are of concern and a source of problems. As you complete the Student-Athlete Challenge #6: Tobacco, Marijuana, and Other Drugs Self-Assessment in Box 8.1, reflect on college students' wide social acceptance of tobacco, marijuana, and other drugs. You have probably been exposed to tobacco, marijuana, and other drugs starting at an early age through the media, in the community, and through your peers. How do you make good decisions about these substances?

We know that among college students (including student-athletes), alcohol and tobacco use are common. Less used but still prevalent is marijuana. Other legal drugs such as stimulants and depressants, although less popular than alcohol, tobacco, and marijuana, are still more widely used than cocaine and heroin. The pressure to use drugs is constant. You are vulnerable to pressure to use even in an environment that you believe is safe and protected.

> *It was a great weekend so far: the parties were more than satisfying and the alcohol was flowing wonderfully. It was late at night and I was sitting in my room. There I was in the same seat I'm always in. There was my roommate in the same seat he is always in. This time there were a few more kids there. Things were going great and then one kid pulls out a green baggy filled with some funky-smelling plant. I quickly realized it was marijuana. At first I was nervous but soon became intrigued and curious. They started wrapping it up like it was some sort of Christmas present, continually calling it a "blunt." They started to smoke it and I immediately became hesitant. The so-called blunt soon got passed to me. I immediately tried to pawn it off on the kid next to me. That did not work out well. My friends started to encourage me to "hit it" but all I could think about was "just say no." They started laughing and I wanted nothing of that. Everyone else was doing it; why not just give it a try. So under all the pressure I hit it. That was not so bad. The next thing I remember is waking up confused, not really clear on what happened the night before. I was scared and disappointed in myself. I just did drugs. I did marijuana.*

Box 8.1. Student-Athlete Challenge #6: *Tobacco, Marijuana, and Other Drugs Self-Assessment*

Directions: Evaluate each statement on a scale of 1 to 5, from 1 being "never" to 5 being "almost always." For each statement evaluate if your behavior adds value (+), is neutral (0), or decreases value (–) of your student-athlete success in regards to your classes and sport.

Statement	Never			Almost Always		Value Added		
	1	2	3	4	5	+	0	–
1. I use illegal drugs.	❏	❏	❏	❏	❏	❏	❏	❏
2. I use tobacco products.	❏	❏	❏	❏	❏	❏	❏	❏
3. I use sleep aids when I'm having a hard time falling asleep.	❏	❏	❏	❏	❏	❏	❏	❏
4. I smoke cigarettes when I drink.	❏	❏	❏	❏	❏	❏	❏	❏
5. I know someone who has been drugged at a party.	❏	❏	❏	❏	❏	❏	❏	❏
6. I have taken a drug test.	❏	❏	❏	❏	❏	❏	❏	❏
7. A teammate has failed a drug test.	❏	❏	❏	❏	❏	❏	❏	❏
8. I have performed poorly on a test or assignment because of drug use.	❏	❏	❏	❏	❏	❏	❏	❏
9. I have tried masking agents.	❏	❏	❏	❏	❏	❏	❏	❏
10. I have tried to quit smoking.	❏	❏	❏	❏	❏	❏	❏	❏
11. I have tried to help a friend or family member quit smoking or chewing tobacco.	❏	❏	❏	❏	❏	❏	❏	❏
12. I feel pressured to use drugs.	❏	❏	❏	❏	❏	❏	❏	❏

As a student-athlete and role model within your school, you need to be aware of the perception and/or message you are sending to your peers, professors, family, and younger athletes who may look up to you. It is your choice whether or not you use substances, and it is possible to have a thriving social life in college without using tobacco, marijuana, or other drugs for recreational and social purposes. This chapter focuses on tobacco, marijuana, and other drugs used and abused on college campuses. As a student-athlete, it is important for you to know the facts about the substances you will encounter at parties, in the dorm, on campus, and in the training room, to help you to make decisions that are the best for you.

Understanding Substance Use

Many students arrive on campus and they soon persuade themselves that tobacco, marijuana, and other drugs are part of everyone's reality. Sometimes this perception pushes them to try drugs just to feel like they are part of the crowd. Most students, however, overestimate the level of substance use among college students. They perceive substance usage to be much higher than it actually is. For example, it is easy to think that everyone is drinking and smoking marijuana on a Saturday night when you hear a loud party going on next door. Contrary to what you may believe, most student-athletes are committed to leading pretty healthy lifestyles.

Another aspect of anyone using any drug (e.g., tobacco, marijuana) is their perception of the risks associated with using drugs. A person's perception is shaped to a large degree by their information of the drug (and if it is accurate) and personal experience (as well as family members' and peers' experience). Compare your answers to the questions in Box 8.2 with those of your friends and teammates. How are your perceptions alike? Where do you differ with your friends? Why are there differences?

Not everyone on campus is smoking cigarettes, chewing tobacco, lighting up joints, making blunts, and taking other drugs, although to read the media and to hear some fellow college students (as well as student-athletes) boast of their experiences you might think otherwise. Usage is happening on campus. As you think about tobacco, marijuana, and other drugs it is important to recognize that their usage is not risk free. There are consequences that are not always understood or seen by many students. As with alcohol usage, problems and consequences are frequently denied.

THINK ABOUT IT ✔

❏ What do you think are the most commonly used substances on your campus? Would you feel less safe if you knew that illicit drugs were heavily used by students on campus?

❏ Why is it important for student-athletes to make healthy decisions regarding substance use? What are some of the consequences of making poor choices?

Box 8.2. How Much Do Student-Athletes Risk Using Tobacco, Marijuana, and Other Drugs?

1. How much do you think student-athletes risk harming themselves (physically or in any other way) if they smoke one or two cigarettes a week?

_____ No risk   _____ Great risk

_____ Slight risk   _____ Moderate risk

2. How much do you think student-athletes risk harming themselves (physically or in any other way) if they smoke one or more packs of cigarettes per day?

_____ No risk   _____ Great risk

_____ Slight risk   _____ Moderate risk

3. How much do you think student-athletes risk harming themselves (physically or in any other way) if they try marijuana once or twice?

_____ No risk   _____ Great risk

_____ Slight risk   _____ Moderate risk

4. How much do you think student-athletes risk harming themselves (physically or in any other way) if they smoke marijuana regularly?

_____ No risk   _____ Great risk

_____ Slight risk   _____ Moderate risk

5. How much do you think student-athletes risk harming themselves (physically or in any other way) if they try cocaine or another illegal drug once or twice?

_____ No risk   _____ Great risk

_____ Slight risk   _____ Moderate risk

6. How much do you think student-athletes risk harming themselves (physically or in any other way) if they use cocaine or another illegal drug regularly?

_____ No risk   _____ Great risk

_____ Slight risk   _____ Moderate risk

Source: Adapted from Monitoring the Future, 2007

Tobacco

Yes, Even Student-Athletes Use Tobacco Products

Many people find it surprising when they discover a particular athlete is a smoker. It is weird that athletes, for whom so much depends on how healthy they are physically, would make it hard for themselves by smoking. Do you ever wonder which athletes you know of might smoke? Tobacco use is common among college students including student-athletes and is not limited to cigarettes. College appears to be a time when many students are trying a range of tobacco products and are in danger of developing lifelong nicotine dependence. Using smokeless tobacco products can lead to nicotine addiction just as cigarettes do, and likewise increase risk of cancers of the mouth and throat, the development of precancerous sores in the mouth, and receding gums, according to the American Cancer Society.

The amount of nicotine within the body depends on the delivery mechanism, dosage, and uptake of the drug (e.g., two cigarettes per hour). Nicotine is addictive. Once in the body, nicotine can cause nervousness and anxiety. It may also increase heart rate, which further complicates the body's ability to maintain homeostasis during exercise. Nicotine can increase blood pressure by vasoconstriction of peripheral vessels. If you hang around with smokers you can suffer from irritated nasal and sinus passages due to secondhand smoke, which may lead to upper respiratory tract infections.

Most students who use tobacco have at least considered quitting. Some may have tried a few times to quit. Since smokers usually try to quit several times before succeeding, additional attempts to stop smoking are considered a sign of commitment to quitting. According to researchers, student-athletes who smoked tended to think that quitting was easier than non-athletes did. Student-athletes underestimate the difficulty associated with cessation. For instance, they may stop smoking during the sports season in which they play but view this as an interruption, not really an opening to quit. Clearly, quitting sooner rather than later has important health consequences. Delaying attempts to quit can increase smokers' likelihood of becoming physically addicted to tobacco.

Okay—Your Friend Wants to Quit

Here's the deal. You have a friend who wants to quit smoking and you're wondering just what you can do to help. Listen up. You can make a big difference. Here are a few suggestions on how to help them successfully quit:

Be understanding. Hardly any smoker will say that they're ready to quit first thing tomorrow. In fact, they will go through several stages when trying to quit. In most cases there's a lot of time spent getting used to the idea, getting ready to do it, and actually getting serious. One way to encourage smokers to take quitting seriously is to help them choose an important quit date. They should pick a date within two weeks of deciding to quit to give them enough time to get ready, but not so far away that they will lose their drive to quit. Suggest that they choose a special day such as their birthday, a holiday, or anti-tobacco day such as the Great American Smokeout. If a significant event is not available within two weeks of their deciding to quit, suggest that they choose a day that they don't have class, especially if they usually smoke in between classes. That way they will already be cigarette-free when they return to class and they will not be as distracted during class. Be careful to not nag or pressure them to choose a date.

Be proactive. Remember, it is your friend who needs to make the decision—but that doesn't mean you can't do a little homework. Scope out some of the cessation programs available on-line or on your campus. Do some research on quitting so that when the subject comes up you'll be ready, willing, and able to lend a hand. For instance, you could ask them to think about the top three most important reasons they would like to quit and/or ask them to name two people besides yourself who could also help them (Box 8.3).

Be supportive. When your friend does decide to take the plunge, be supportive. Chances are the withdrawal symptoms will make them into someone you don't even want to hang with! They may be cranky, anxious, or just plain difficult. Common feelings of smoking withdrawal include:

- Feeling depressed

- Not being able to sleep

STUDENT REFLECTION

Box 8.3. What Are Your Three Most Important Reasons for Wanting to Quit?

1. _____

_____

2. _____

_____

3. _____

_____

Two people I can call to help me:

Name _____ Phone _____

Name _____ Phone _____

- Getting cranky, frustrated, or mad

- Feeling anxious, nervous, or restless

- Having trouble thinking clearly

- Feeling hungry or gaining weight

But hang in there, these symptoms will pass—usually in a few days. And remember, don't take the emotional ups and downs personally—they are not your fault. Instead, help them think about certain things that trigger, or turn on, their need for a cigarette and how they will handle these situations. These triggers can be moods, feelings, places, or things they do. Knowing and recording these triggers in a craving journal can help them stay in control (Box 8.4).

Finally, since weight gain is a worry and common side effect of quitting, encourage your friend to choose the many tasty and healthy products now on the market, like no-salt pretzels

STUDENT REFLECTION

Box 8.4. Can You Overcome Cravings?

Craving Journal   Date: _____

Cigarette #	Time	Craving level Low = 1 High = 5	Location	Who I was with	Feelings
Example # 1	10:45 a.m.	4	in dorm room	alone	stressed out
1					
2					
3					
4					
5					
6					
7					
8					

Adapted from *One Step at a Time Program—Book 3.* Toronto, Ontario: Canadian Cancer Society, 1998.

or popcorn, and offer to work out with them at the gym, especially since they will be able to breathe easier. Remind them that the good news is that most ex-smokers will lose most of the weight they gained without doing anything.

Be thoughtful. If you smoke, try not to smoke around your friend. When you do things together, suggest doing an activity that doesn't include smoking and try hanging out in places where smoking is not allowed, like malls, movie theaters, or restaurants. A few other actions may help your friend:

- Make things clean and fresh at home and in their car by cleaning drapes and clothes. Buy flowers for them and remind them that they will now be able to enjoy their scent more as their sense of smell returns.

- Throw away all cigarettes and matches. Give or throw away lighters and ashtrays. Remember the ashtray and lighter in the car!

- Some smokers save one pack of cigarettes "just in case" or because they want to prove they have the willpower not to smoke. Don't let them! Saving one pack just makes it easier to start smoking again.

Be there. Helping your friend to stay tobacco free can be a challenge. It's a fact: lots of people trying to quit will relapse. Two things tend to happen when people have a cigarette after quitting. First, they think that all is lost, that there is no point in trying any longer. It is like the dieter who has that first piece of cake: "I have blown my diet, so I may as well finish the cake." Thinking like that only gets you into more trouble. An entire cake is worse than one slice, and a pack of cigarettes is worse than one puff. The second thing that happens after a cigarette is that smokers tend to feel guilty and depressed. They tend to beat themselves up. This makes them feel worse. This leads to an even greater urge to smoke, and then they often keep smoking. The thing to remember is to not come down too hard on them. Just remind them of the reasons they wanted to quit in the first place and the progress they've made so far, and encourage them to try again if they relapse. The bottom line is, just be there for them.

Encouragement and Support to Quit

Everybody knows that withdrawal comes with the territory of quitting, but that doesn't make it any easier. It can be hard and even frustrating for the person quitting to deal with withdrawal and for those around the person. But understanding what's going on, physically and psychologically, can help and can assist you in helping a friend quit.

- When smokers quit, they begin to go through some changes, some physical, some emotional. The physical symptoms, while annoying and difficult, are not life threatening. Replacement products such as the patch or gum can help reduce many of these physical symptoms. For most smokers, the bigger challenge is the psychological part of quitting.

- This psychological part of smoking is really hard to beat because smoking becomes linked to so many things—things like waking up in the morning, eating, reading, watching television, drinking coffee, and so on. It's like a ritual. Your body becomes used to having a hit with certain activities and will miss this link when you first become smoke free.

- It will take time to "unlink" smoking from these activities. Unfortunately, smoking substitutes can't relieve the psychological need to smoke. That's why it's so important for the smoker to create a plan to deal with situations that trigger their urge to smoke. Smokers can also ask friends and family for support with simple things like walking around the building before class instead of smoking, and when a smoker goes through withdrawal, they need to keep this in mind. Even though they may not act like themselves, and they may feel rotten, remind them these feelings will pass. After thirty days or so of not smoking, this will all be behind them.

In the meantime, here are some of the withdrawal symptoms smokers may experience and what they can do about them. Share them with your friend.

- *Craving*—This is the body's physical addiction saying, "I need a hit now!" Each craving will last for only a couple of minutes and these will eventually stop happening altogether in about seven days. Smokers can use tobacco replacement products to help reduce cravings. If the smoker still feels the urge, they can admit out loud to themselves or someone else that they are having a craving. Then they should count to one hundred and let the feeling pass—and it will, usually within a couple of minutes. Additionally, they can use their craving journal to record emotions related to cravings and figure out how to handle these same situations better in the future.

- *Difficulty concentrating*—"Help, I quit smoking and I can't concentrate!" Some people say nicotine helps focus their attention. When they quit smoking, the increased blood flow and oxygen can lead to a feeling of mental fogginess. If this happens, they should try making lists and daily schedules to keep organized, and then set aside some total relaxation time when they don't have to concentrate on anything.

- *Fatigue/sleeping problems*—Trouble sleeping and fatigue are common symptoms of withdrawal. Because nicotine increases one's metabolism to an abnormally high rate, when people stop smoking their metabolism drops back to normal, making them feel like their energy level has dropped. So what can they do? They need to get their body used to the new metabolic rate by getting plenty of sleep whenever possible. Although sleep patterns may be interrupted at first, this is normal and temporary.

- *Irritability*—If you have snapped at someone after quitting or had a new nonsmoker snap at you, you know what we are talking about. Irritability is caused by the body trying to adjust to the sudden disappearance of all those chemicals it's been used to. The best way to handle this is for smokers to simply be honest with those around them that they are trying to quit and they do not feel like themselves.

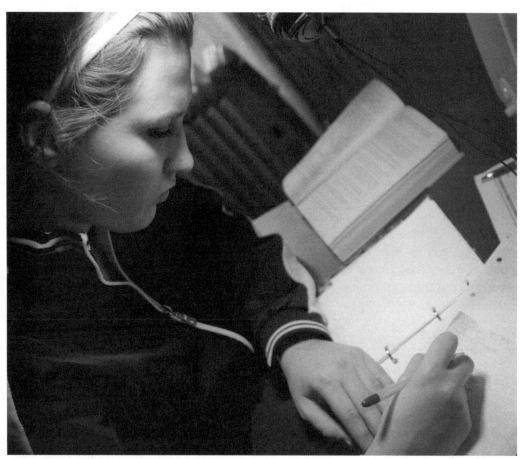
© Alexander Motrenko/ShutterStock, Inc.

Sometimes your friend will not be able to fight the urge to smoke. Again, if they do slip up, try to convince them that it is not a failure. Instead, tell them that successful quitters use behavioral and mental coping skills when they have an urge. For example, some behavioral coping skills include actions like leaving a stressful situation, chewing gum, calling a friend, or going for a walk. Mental coping skills include taking a deep breath, thinking about how much progress they have made so far, and thinking about what smoking does to their health.

Think of it as a lapse in concentration and help them renew their commitment to quit. It is a good idea to remind them that you are confident that they are capable of not smoking. In addition, encourage them to reward themselves in new ways. One good suggestion is for them to give themselves a gift at the end of each week or month that they were successful in fulfilling their commitment to not smoking. Help them calculate the amount of money they usually

THINK ABOUT IT

❑ How can you best help and support a teammate who is trying to quit smoking or chewing tobacco? Brainstorm a few ideas to help them cope with stressful athletic and academic pressures in a healthier and more productive way than by using tobacco.

❑ List the kinds of tobacco education you have received over the years either in school, through sports, or in your community. What impact did these programs have on you?

spend during the time period on buying cigarettes and try to match the cost of the gift with this amount. Suggest that they keep a record of these expenses in a notebook to record their gifts and costs. For example, in week one, they could spend $25 on a movie and snacks for two people rather than spend that money on cigarettes.

Marijuana

Addictive, Controversial, Illegal

Lots of people think that smoking marijuana is harmless and they do not have to quit something that is not harming their bodies. Like tobacco, marijuana is highly addictive and problematic for student-athletes. Marijuana is the most commonly abused illicit drug in the United States. A dry, shredded green/brown mix of flowers, stems, seeds, and leaves of the hemp plant *Cannabis sativa,* it is usually smoked as a cigarette (joint, nail) or in a pipe (bong). It also is smoked in blunts, which are cigars that have been emptied of tobacco and refilled with marijuana, often in combination with another drug. It might also be mixed in food or brewed as a tea. As a more concentrated, resinous form it is called hashish and, as a sticky black liquid, hash oil. Marijuana smoke has a pungent, distinctive, usually sweet-and-sour odor. There are countless street terms for marijuana including pot, herb, weed, grass, widow, ganja, and hash, as well as terms derived from trademarked varieties of cannabis, such as Bubble Gum, Northern Lights, Fruity Juice, Afghani #1, and a number of Skunk varieties. College students report that they get marijuana by buying it, trading something else for it, getting it for free or sharing someone else's, or growing it.

Although marijuana is potentially less addictive than other drugs, such as cocaine, crack, heroin, and barbiturates, it remains one of the few drugs that is controversial. It is difficult to wade through the emotion and politics to tease out the objective clinical reality. The potency of marijuana is determined by the percentage of its active ingredient, THC (tetrahydrocannabinol). Scientists have learned a great deal about how THC acts in the brain to produce its many effects. When someone smokes marijuana, THC passes rapidly from the lungs into the bloodstream, which carries the chemical to organs throughout the body, including the brain. In the brain, THC connects to specific sites called *cannabinoid receptors* on nerve cells and thereby influences the activity of those cells. Some brain areas have many cannabinoid receptors; others have few or none. Many cannabinoid receptors are found in the parts of the brain that influence pleasure, memory, thought, concentration, sensory and time perception, and coordinated movement.

The physiological effects of smoking marijuana include poor concentration and psychomotor problems that can last up to twenty-four hours. This means that marijuana can interfere with your effectiveness during practice or a game, even several hours after usage. The biggest effects are on hand-eye coordination, reaction time, tracking ability, and perceptual accuracy, which can make it difficult for you to catch, throw, or kick a ball. Other physical effects of smoking marijuana include wheezing when you exercise, increasing your heart rate, and decreasing your workload capacity. Unlike alcohol, marijuana's physiological effects stay in the body for a long time. For regular users, THC can stay in one's body for up to a month. For non-regular users, it is eliminated from the body in about five to seven days.

The bottom line for college student-athletes is that it is a banned substance that does impact mental and physical performance. However, that does not stop student-athletes from using it. And you are aware that from urine to hair to sweat to blood to saliva, a multitude of ways exist to detect marijuana. There are many techniques floating around for flushing your body free of drugs or tricking the tests by loading up on herbs, certain foods, magic detoxifier pills, coffee, and so on. You may have heard about spiking your specimen with adulterants. But many of these techniques are myths. For example, there is speculation that loading up on water before a urine drug test might dilute drugs and metabolites just enough to put them below the cutoff levels. However, lots of water makes your urine look pale. It's a healthy sign that you're well hydrated, but it's also a waving flag that you might have tried to "flush." NORML (National Organization for the Reform of Marijuana Laws) suggests that you might be able to beat watery-urine detection "visually" if you also take vitamin B-2, which tints your urine yellow.

Drug testing has become a part of American life, giving rise to a multibillion-dollar-per-year industry that exists solely to break the body into measurable pieces and detail your private life for the benefit of your school, team, and sport. Remember, marijuana is by far the most widely used illicit drug and therefore the most widely detected substance in drug testing. Twenty-five million Americans smoked pot last year, and THC stays in the body for a relatively long time compared to other drugs, two factors that make marijuana the ideal target for the drug-test market. And although people never believe that they will get caught, with year-round NCAA drug testing, student-athletes can harm their scholastic and athletic careers with the use of marijuana.

Box 8.5. What Have You Learned About Marijuana?

Below are five common myths about marijuana and its usage. Disprove each myth by citing facts you have learned in this chapter about marijuana.

Myth 1: Marijuana is harmless. It's no worse for you than smoking cigarettes.

Myth 2: Marijuana is not addictive.

Myth 3: Youth experimentation with marijuana is inevitable. It's no big deal to try it once.

Myth 4: Marijuana is not associated with violence as with drugs like cocaine and heroin.

Myth 5: Drug tests are not effective at detecting marijuana.

Do I Have a Marijuana Problem?

The concern for student-athletes (as well as for anyone) who uses marijuana is that at some point marijuana use can control your life. You lose interest in all else; your dreams go up in smoke. Like any other addiction, your life, thinking, and desires center around marijuana—scoring it, dealing it, and finding ways to stay high. Marijuana was once thought to be a gateway to other illicit drug use, but researchers have not found conclusive evidence to support this claim. Many people simply use and abuse only marijuana. Many student-athletes may want to quit because they are tired of worrying about getting caught, being thrown off the team, and perhaps losing their athletic scholarship.

Quitting the use of marijuana is not easy. Most people do not just stop. Similar to smoking, it requires a conscientious effort, plan, and quit date. You need to build support and resources to help with the cravings, frustrations, and anxiety. Many people find the twelve questions developed by Marijuana Anonymous helpful in reflecting about the role of marijuana in their lives:

1. Has using pot stopped being fun?

2. Do you ever get high alone?

3. Is it hard for you to imagine a life without marijuana?

4. Do you find that your friends are determined by your marijuana use?

5. Do you smoke marijuana to avoid dealing with your problems?

6. Do you smoke pot to cope with your feelings?

7. Does your marijuana use let you live in a privately defined world?

8. Have you ever failed to keep promises you made about cutting down or controlling your dope smoking?

9. Has your use of marijuana caused problems with memory, concentration, or motivation?

10. When your stash is nearly empty, do you feel anxious or worried about how to get more?

11. Do you plan your life around your marijuana use?

12. Have friends or relatives ever complained that your pot smoking is damaging your relationship with them? (Source: Marijuana Anonymous Web site, http://www.marijuana-anonymous. org/Pages/12quest.html)

If you answered yes to any of the above questions, you may have a problem with marijuana and should consider quitting. Once a person has decided to quit, like cigarettes, it's time to pick the all-important Quit Date. Make sure it's pretty soon—like maybe in the next month. Again, choosing a date too far in the future will make it easier to rationalize a way out of it, but there also needs to be enough time to prepare. Then it's time to come up with a solid plan. Treat yourself by finding support on campus. Ask a trusted friend for support. Try to find resources on campus where you can talk with someone who can help you figure out how to stop using marijuana as well as not relapse once you have stopped. Go to Chapter 11 and read the sections on finding support on campus. You work hard and deserve a marijuana- (as well as tobacco-) free life.

THINK ABOUT IT

❑ Identify at least three ways that the use of marijuana can negatively affect a person's athletic performance.

❑ What would you do if you knew a teammate was using marijuana regularly? Would you confront him or her about it? Why or why not?

❑ List the consequences that an athlete could face if he or she was caught abusing marijuana or any other substance. How would these consequences impact the season, team spirit, and/or his or her future?

Other Drugs and Student-Athletes

Living Drug Free

It often seems like student-athletes are constantly having to make decisions about their use of alcohol, tobacco, marijuana, pain medications (NSAIDs and prescriptions), and ergogenic aids. Managing these decisions is a chore. To add to the stress and strain are other drugs that are common and available to student-athletes. Some are prescription medications that are legal but misused and abused. Others are illicit (illegal) drugs. All of the drugs have the potential to be addictive and destructive to your athletic and academic careers. However, given their strong attraction, the threat of hurting your career may not be enough to dissuade use. Probably the best defense is to be aware of the drugs and to get support to avoid their use—including experimental or occasional use.

Depressants

Depressants, also known as sedatives or "downers," are substances that slow down the functioning of the central nervous system. As a result, reaction time, muscle reflex, judgment, and coordination become impaired. Alcohol is a depressant and is by far the most used and abused depressant among student-athletes. However, it is not the only one. Depressants include barbiturates, tranquilizers, and sedative-hypnotics, such as the "date rape" drug. Barbiturates are anti-anxiety drugs that depress the central nervous system to the point that the user drops off to sleep. They act much like an anesthetic. Student-athletes are under tremendous stress and may turn to barbiturates to help them relax and fall asleep at night. The use of barbiturates is dangerous because student-athletes who use them may slip into a vicious cycle in which they become dependent on "downers" to help them sleep, and then "uppers" to get going again in the morning. Likewise, not following prescribed dosage or mixing use with alcohol or other substances is dangerous.

A type of depressant found on college campuses is sedative-hypnotic drugs, also known as "date rape" drugs. These drugs produce a drunk-like or sleepy state that can last for hours. They include Rohypnol and GHB (gamma-hydroxybutyrate). Rohypnol is also known as R-2, roofies, roophies, and roaches. Rohypnol has no odor, color, or taste. It usually comes in a pill form but sometimes can be a powder. Because you can't see, taste, or smell the drug, it's very easy to be fooled by it. GHB is a clear liquid. It can be mistaken for water because it is usually found in a small (30 ml) clear plastic bottle, a water bottle, or even a GatorAde bottle, which contains several doses. One quick taste and you'll know it's not water. It is also found as a white powder, but this is not as common.

People often slip these drugs into the drinks of unsuspecting students. It makes a person feel very relaxed, confused, and spaced out. It can also make a person not able to move or talk. Too much of the drug can make a person pass out or slip into a coma. Hours after the drug has worn off, the person usually has little or no memory of what happened. Combined with alcohol these drugs can be deadly.

People will slip the drug into a person's drink without them knowing it just to take advantage of them sexually. The abuser will wait until the victim is too out of it to say "no" and will have sex with them.

A person can do several things to protect themselves from the date rape drug. Here are just a few:

- Don't let anyone fix you a drink. Always pour your own.

- Travel with a group of people and stick together at a party.

- Stay sober. Don't use drugs or alcohol, so you have a clear head at all times.

Look out not only for yourself, but also for your friends. A really good idea is to not let your friends get too drunk or wasted. If they do party too hard, take them home and stay with them to make sure they are okay. Don't let them disappear and don't let them wander off with a member of the opposite sex.

Hallucinogens

Hallucinogens are substances that produce hallucinations, or perceived distortions of reality. Marijuana is a hallucinogen. The category also includes LSD (lysergic acid diethylamide), PCP (phencyclidine), "Special K" (ketamine), Ecstasy, psilocybin ("magic" mushrooms), and peyote (mescaline). Someone who uses a hallucinogen may feel a higher awareness of sensory input and an enhanced sense of clarity or clearness and diminished control over what is experienced. In general, hallucinogens distort reality and heighten sensation. These drugs do not typically produce a physical dependence, but users can become psychologically dependent. Although hallucinogenic drugs generally produce euphoric feelings and sensations, there are serious downsides associated with their usage such as acute anxiety and panic reactions, depression, mood swings, and distortions in body images. Hallucinogens cause pupil dilation, increased body temperature and blood pressure, increases in heartbeat and reflexes, tremors, nausea, vomiting, diarrhea, and loss of appetite. Generally, it is unlikely that student-athletes would abuse hallucinogens to enhance athletic performance, but they might use them recreationally as a way to cope with stressors. Student-athletes who try hallucinogenic substances tend to think that they have no effect on their performance and skills. They view the usage of hallucinogens, such as marijuana, as purely recreational. Unfortunately, the effects of using these social drugs carry over to their play.

Stimulants

Stimulants or "uppers" are substances that excite or increase the activity of the central nervous system and so increase heart rate, blood pressure, and the rate of brain function. Earlier we discussed the stimulants caffeine (Chapter 6) and nicotine (in the current chapter). Discussed in this section are the stimulants cocaine and amphetamines. While most stimulants make a user psychologically dependent quite quickly, they are unlikely to make the person physically dependent when judged by life-threatening withdrawal symptoms. Many student-athletes have attempted to improve their physical performance by trying stimulants.

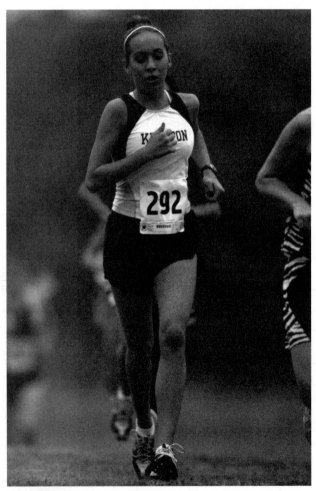

© Shawn Pecor/ShutterStock, Inc.

Cocaine is a stimulant that can be abused by athletes and can lead to dependency. It is an illicit drug. Its use and possession are illegal. Cocaine usage in sports dates back to the late 1800s, when cyclists combined this substance with opiate drugs to enhance their performance during endurance races. Today, cocaine has reemerged in sports headlines as several high-profile athletes have abused this illegal substance for recreational purposes. Although cocaine's effects may not be long lasting, because it enters and leaves the central nervous system quickly, the physical distress is extremely dangerous. For example, cocaine increases heart rate, constricts blood vessels, enhances the supply of glucose and lipid in the circulation, and dilates the bronchioles. Some athletes believe that the elevation of heart rate and circulation may enhance their performance and athletic stamina; unfortunately, this is a misconception. It speeds up the processes of the nervous system and disturbs the heartbeat to the point that it affects the brain, may trigger the onset of seizures, and may result in death.

Another performance-supporting stimulant is amphetamine. Amphetamines are prescription drugs often misused. The drugs are used by athletes to keep going during intense exercise. They allow athletes to perform past the normal point of fatigue, particularly when performance is down because of fatigue or lack of sleep. Amphetamines have an effect similar to that of cocaine, but the effects are more dramatic. The substance enters the brain quickly and increases alertness. People on amphetamine are talkative, energetic, and move around a lot. This substance increases heart rate, raises blood pressure, dilates bronchioles, and increases glucose and fatty acids in the bloodstream. Amphetamines are effective at giving the athlete that extra burst of energy just before competition, but that boost comes at a very high price. At high doses, amphetamines increase heart rate and blood pressure to dangerous levels. In addition, as the substance is eliminated from the body, the athlete "crashes" into exhaustion, and performance is drastically reduced. As a result, many student-athletes get caught in a trap where they need more amphetamines to recover from their crash. The substance is extremely addictive. Amphetamines are dangerous both psychologically and physically because they do provide short-term positive reinforcing effects on performance, such as improved concentration, alertness, and endurance. Many athletes are enticed by the possible physical gains that are associated with amphetamines and therefore the potential for abuse becomes high.

Many student-athletes are lured into trying stimulants because of preconceived notions that they will provide a quick way to make significant gains in strength and endurance in a short amount of time. Many student-athletes think that the stimulants will give them a competitive advantage that they cannot achieve on their own. For example, a long-distance runner may need to shave a few minutes off his time to qualify for nationals. The day of his qualifying race, he may decide to use an amphetamine to give his body a boost. The runner may tell himself that he will use the stimulant only this one time. Once he qualifies for nationals, he will go back to training harder and more frequently to improve his time. Unfortunately, it is harder than he realized to try a substance just one time. The athlete may run well in the qualifying race, but shortly after he crosses the finish line, he crashes. The following morning he cannot even generate enough energy to get through practice. Soon he is relying on caffeine to stay awake and he begins popping pills to keep his body going. Before he realizes it, he is spiraling out of control. He is jittery, irritable, and unable to focus. By the day of the national championship, the athlete's body is in poor shape to compete. He is dehydrated and lacking the nutrients he needs to perform.

Narcotics

The term "narcotic," derived from the Greek word for stupor, originally referred to a variety of substances that dulled the senses and relieved pain. Today the term is used in a number of ways. Some individuals define narcotics as those substances that bind at opiate receptors (cellular membrane proteins activated by substances like heroin or morphine) while others refer to any illicit substance as a narcotic. Confusing is that cocaine and coca leaves are also classified as "narcotics" in the Controlled Substances Act (CSA). These substances neither bind opiate receptors nor produce morphine-like effects, and they are discussed in the section on stimulants. The use of narcotics therapeutically to treat pain was discussed in Chapter 4. Narcotics are administered in a variety of ways. Some are taken orally, taken transdermally (skin patches), or injected. They are also available as suppositories. As drugs of abuse, they are often smoked, sniffed, or injected. Drug effects depend heavily on the dose, route of administration, and previous exposure to the drug. Aside from their medical use, narcotics produce a general sense of well-being by reducing tension, anxiety, and aggression. These effects are helpful in a therapeutic setting but contribute to their abuse.

Narcotic use is associated with a variety of unwanted effects including drowsiness, inability to concentrate, apathy, lessened physical activity, constriction of the pupils, dilation of the subcutaneous blood vessels causing flushing of the face and neck, constipation, nausea and vomiting, and most significantly, respiratory depression. As the dose is increased, the subjective, analgesic (pain relief), and toxic effects become more pronounced. Except in cases of acute intoxication, there is no loss of motor coordination or slurred speech as occurs with many depressants.

Inhalants

Although a lot of effort has appropriately been focused on talking about illicit drugs such as marijuana, cocaine, and LSD, often ignored are the dangers posed to people from common household products that contain volatile solvents or aerosols. Products such as glues, nail polish remover, lighter fluid, spray paints, deodorant and hair sprays, whipped cream canisters, and cleaning fluids are widely available. Many people inhale the vapors from these sources in search of quick intoxication without being aware of the serious health consequences that can result.

Nearly all abused products produce effects similar to anesthetics, which slow down the body's function. Varying upon level of dosage, the user can experience slight stimulation, a feeling of less inhibition, or loss of consciousness. The user can also suffer from sudden sniffing death syndrome: the user can die the first, tenth, or one hundredth time he or she uses an inhalant.

THINK ABOUT IT

- ❏ Often student-athletes say things like, "I had four cups of coffee this morning just to stay awake during class," or "I took No-Doz last night to stay up and cram for a final." What tips could you offer these students so that they would not have to rely on stimulants?

- ❏ What are some common reasons why you or a teammate would abuse a substance? Which group of substances (stimulants, depressants, hallucinogens, narcotics, inhalants) do you think are most used by athletes? Rank them in the order that you believe they are used by athletes from most used to least used.

- ❏ How does the use of depressants by student-athletes lead to abuse of other substances?

PLUGGED IN TO SPORTS

Student-Athletes and Technology

As a society we are driven by mass media. Think of the amount of time we spend watching television or movies, listening to the radio, or working at the computer. Mass media have a huge influence on our choices, awareness, and behavior; just look at the effect of marketing and advertisements! Major cigarette companies spend billions of dollars each year on advertising.

One of the most pervasive and sustained images in the media is that college students will inevitably drink, smoke, and do drugs. This image is perpetuated by advertising, media messages, and sports events in which beer/alcohol sponsorship is evident and specific, as well as by tobacco-related promotions for particular times of the academic year, such as spring break. Simply "blaming the media" for fueling us with misperceptions is too simplistic; the answer lies in developing media literacy or identifying the meaning of the media images. Media literacy is the ability to "read" television, radio, Internet, and print advertisements, and other mass media. As a consumer, you should be aware of the four elements often referred to as the marketing mix or the "4Ps" of marketing: product, placement, pricing, and the product promotion to you the buyer. So, next time you consider buying something, think of the 4Ps and how relevant they are to your purchase.

Chapter Summary

As a student-athlete, there is a good chance you've already been offered a wide range of drugs. If it has not happened yet, it will. These drugs may be legal or illegal. You may find the idea seductive, because you hear that they can boost your performance, help you have a good time, or help you fit in with the in-crowd. So, it is important for you to educate yourself and become aware of possible substance reactions, and how they can affect you now and later.

Many student-athletes abuse substances because of stressors in their life. These stressors can be physical, such as pulled tendons, exhaustion from a strenuous workout or game, and other athletic challenges. Or, stressors can be emotional, as when you try to keep up with your athletic performance, classroom assignments, and just possibly your self-image as a well-known campus star. Despite the evidence that drugs really don't help your athletic performance, some student-athletes continue to use them.

Often the student-athletes that abuse substances are abusing the substances to enhance their performance or get their edge back, particularly if an athlete was more successful in high school and now in college may be on the second or third string of players. They may hope that these substances will increase strength and endurance to help them play through the pain of an injury. As we have discussed, this is not true and instead can cause a lot of harm to the body.

Furthermore, student-athletes who use drugs recreationally do it to feel good and experience altered states of consciousness. There can be a lot of pressure to "join the crowd" at parties, and student-athletes may feel under particular social pressure to do this. In addition, student-athletes are natural competitors, not likely to pass up a dare. They may believe that being in excellent physical shape will reduce or eliminate any negative effects from the drugs. All of this is potentially a recipe for disaster, and as a responsible teammate, you need to educate yourself and other players on the nature and effects of substance abuse.

Student-athletes encounter a variety of different individuals, each with their own social and recreational patterns. Because it is important that athletes work closely with their teammates, it is also important that student-athletes know how to recognize and assist teammates who are in social or physical situations that may become dangerous, unhealthy, or troubling. The best way to help a fellow teammate is by preventing them from getting into a harmful situation in the first place. A proactive approach is to create a positive environment within your team. Because peers have much more of an effect on students than coaches, doctors, or other adults, a peer can be a great role model and source of support. As a student-athlete, you can relate to stressors that your fellow teammates are experiencing and can be a positive influence, promoting healthy living and providing accurate drug and alcohol information. Open dialogue among team members regarding tobacco, marijuana, and other drug use can help everyone understand and identify problem behaviors and make healthy decisions.

Your Thoughts

1. Read this scenario and respond to the question below:

   The basketball team has a zero-tolerance drug policy. Anyone caught doing illegal drugs will be kicked off the team. There is a party on campus and a group of people are smoking marijuana. The party gets busted by campus security, and four students who were seen smoking marijuana are taken to the campus police office. The four students are let go by campus police with just a warning. One of the students was the star forward on the basketball team. The next day, the news about the party and four students being taken away by campus police was all over campus. The basketball coach hears of the story and is faced with a tough decision. If you were the coach, how would you handle this situation? Why?

2. Marijuana is the most widely used illicit drug in America, and there has been debate over the years about whether or not the substance should be legalized. List three reasons that people might give for why marijuana should be legalized. List three reasons why marijuana should not be legalized. What are the consequences of legalizing marijuana? In your opinion, should marijuana be legalized? Why?

3. How do you educate your fellow college student-athletes about tobacco, marijuana, and other drug facts and myths?

CHAPTER
9

Challenge #7: Sex and Relationships

Learning Objectives

After completing this chapter, you will be able to:

- *Identify tips and methods for safe sex*

- *Identify different types of sexually transmitted diseases*

- *Understand sexual assault and rape and have an understanding of how to protect yourself from these sorts of incidents*

- *Discuss sexual orientation and the importance of acceptance and understanding*

- *Understand the dangers and repercussions of sexual harassment*

© Photos.com

Student-Athletes Say:

- My ex-boyfriend always told me what to think and what to do. He wanted to make all my decisions for me. He would also always get really mad when I wanted to hang out with my friends instead of him. At the time, I felt I had no choice but to listen to him because I didn't want him to break up with me.

- While in high school and living at home, I would never have dreamed about looking at porn on the Internet. There were just some limits in my house that you knew you could not cross.

- I've heard about other college students contracting sexually transmitted diseases, but I assumed it would never happen to me. I'm usually careful, but there have been a few times that I have had unprotected sex. I worry that I may have contracted something and I don't even know where to get tested or if it is confidential.

- I constantly hear people on campus referring to female athletes as dykes or lesbians. I really take offense to comments like this because they're untrue, and stereotypes like this just make it more difficult for people to be comfortable with themselves.

- I hear that abstinence is the most effective contraception, but it's just unrealistic. My girlfriend is taking birth control, but I am unclear about the best way to protect myself from getting an STD.

- I hear a lot of guys in the locker room talking about their sexual experiences. The way they talk about girls makes me really uncomfortable. They make me feel like a loser because I'm not going out every night looking to score.

- At my school, girls flock around the football players like we're celebrities. We call them "groupies." They show up at all our games and parties, and they're always willing to hook up.

Student-athletes can experience difficulty talking openly about sexual matters. This lack of communication contributes to the perpetuation of myths and misinformation about sexuality despite the fact that the media give increased attention to all aspects of sexual behavior. Almost nothing is unmentionable in the popular media or on the Internet. The Internet in particular has opened the door to sexual material to anyone with Internet access. Yet this increased knowledge regarding sexual behavior and sexuality does not appear to have resulted in encouraging people to talk more freely about their own sexual concerns, nor has it reduced their anxiety about sexuality. For many student-athletes (as for a lot of people) sex remains a delicate topic, and they find it difficult to communicate their sexual wants, especially to a person close to them.

Some students (including student-athletes) become sexually active for the first time during college because they have more freedom, opportunity, and a desire to explore and experiment. Likewise, some students (including student-athletes) have become sexually active in high school and come to college with information and experience. One of the goals for this chapter is to help you value your sexuality and find answers to questions or concerns related to your sexuality. Many student-athletes experience needless guilt, shame, worries, and inhibition merely because they keep their questions and concerns about sexuality secret. Moreover, keeping your questions and concerns to yourself can hinder your efforts to determine your own values regarding sex. Likewise, the reality of HIV/AIDS challenges sexually active individuals to rethink their sexual behavior.

This chapter will refresh your memory on many important issues regarding the exploration of your sexuality during college and beyond. The chapter aims to answer some of the common questions many college students may have about sex. As you complete the Student-Athlete Challenge #7: Sex and Relationships Self-Assessment in Box 9.1, consider your beliefs, orientation, and experiences. How do you navigate the sexual relations and aspects of your life within an environment with freedom and opportunity to explore your sexuality?

Being a college student-athlete complicates the sexual lives of many individuals due to two concerns. First, student-athletes value their physical abilities, which often translate into other people being sexually interested and attracted to them. Second, there are myths and misconceptions about student-athletes' sexual abilities and entitlement to engage in sexual activities, void of feelings, emotions, and meaningful relationships, simply because they are athletes. These two concerns can make your life more complicated and potentially your relationships and sexual behavior more visible than your fellow college students'. It is another source of stress in your life. The following situation could easily happen to any college student-athlete:

> I was really interested in Joe, and one night after our match I saw him at a party. Both of us were drinking a lot to celebrate winning championship doubles, and we really hit it off. By the end of the night we were both a little drunk. He ended up walking me home, and we had sex. I guess I was more intoxicated than I thought, or maybe I was just caught up in the moment, but regardless, we did not use a condom. The next day, he was so insensitive; all he wanted to know was if I was on the pill, and thankfully I was. What a relief, I was safe.
>
> The next day in the locker room after practice, a few of my teammates were asking me about my wild evening. They saw him walking me home the night before, and they wanted to know what happened. I told them that he stayed over. They started to snicker and make their usual crude comments. Then, my friend Cindy said, "I hope you

Box 9.1. Student-Athlete Challenge #7: *Sex and Relationships*
Self-Assessment

Directions: Evaluate each statement on a scale of 1 to 5, from 1 being "never" to 5 being "almost always." For each statement evaluate if your behavior adds value (+), is neutral (0), or decreases value (−) in regard to your student-athlete success in your classes and sport.

Statement	Never				Almost Always	Value Added		
	1	2	3	4	5	+	0	−
1. Sex and sexuality are topics of conversation in the locker room.	❑	❑	❑	❑	❑	❑	❑	❑
2. I read up on STDs, HIV, and other diseases including causes, symptoms, and treatments.	❑	❑	❑	❑	❑	❑	❑	❑
3. I engage in sexual activities that are unprotected.	❑	❑	❑	❑	❑	❑	❑	❑
4. I participate in sex conversations and even exaggerate my own sexual stories.	❑	❑	❑	❑	❑	❑	❑	❑
5. I am uncomfortable having a gay teammate.	❑	❑	❑	❑	❑	❑	❑	❑
6. I have more than one sexual partner at a time.	❑	❑	❑	❑	❑	❑	❑	❑
7. I have been tested for STDs.	❑	❑	❑	❑	❑	❑	❑	❑
8. I am comfortable discussing sexual activity with my peers and/or my partner.	❑	❑	❑	❑	❑	❑	❑	❑
9. I feel pressured by my peers to be sexually active.	❑	❑	❑	❑	❑	❑	❑	❑
10. I go with my instincts regarding people I meet and situations I am placed in.	❑	❑	❑	❑	❑	❑	❑	❑
11. I have been in situations where an individual has made unwanted sexual advances toward me.	❑	❑	❑	❑	❑	❑	❑	❑
12. I am sexually active.	❑	❑	❑	❑	❑	❑	❑	❑

used protection, Joe gets around." I told her to back off, and I assumed her comment was just more immature "trash talk." When I got home from practice, I started to worry. What if I did contract an STD? I was too embarrassed to ask my teammates, and I certainly did not want to go to the Campus Health Center because everyone would see me.

Sexuality is part of your personhood and should not be thought of as an activity divorced from your feelings, values, and relationships. Although childhood and adolescent experiences do have an impact on shaping your present attitudes toward sex and your sexual behavior, you are in a position to modify your attitudes and behavior if you are not satisfied with yourself as a sexual being. Developing your own sexual views, you need to evaluate your own sexual attitudes and become aware of the myths and misconceptions you may harbor. Another important step in developing your sexual views is learning to be open in talking about sexual concerns, including your fears and desires, with at least one other person you trust.

Understanding Your Sexuality

Sexual experiences can be among life's most fulfilling experiences; however, there are also risks and negative factors associated with them. Relationships are complicated, and when they become sexual, they are even more complex. Whether you are currently sexually active or not, you may have questions and it is important to get the facts. Learning the facts about sex is a good way to answer tough questions, make intelligent choices, and protect you or your partner from accidental pregnancy, sexually transmitted diseases, and emotional problems. Furthermore, you can and should decide what sexual practices are acceptable for you, and this decision making is enhanced when you are able to explore sexual issues without needless guilt or shame. It is important that your sexual behavior be consistent with your value system.

A part of understanding your sexuality is to know your body and what is "normal" for you, so that you can tell when something is different. If you are a woman, you need to monitor the length of your menstrual periods, the amount of blood, and level of discomfort. Being aware of how your body normally functions will help you know if anything changes or if you develop any symptoms that signal pregnancy or a sexually transmitted disease. Similarly, men need to be aware of their bodies and check themselves for skin changes, such as bumps or sores, on the genitals, discharge from the penis, or discomfort when urinating, as these could be signs of a sexually transmitted disease.

For both genders sexuality involves sensual experiences. Sensuality implies a full awareness of and sensitivity to the pleasures of sight, sound, smell, taste, and touch. We can all enjoy sensuality without being sexual; sensuality does not have to lead to sexual activity. Nevertheless, sensuality is important in enhancing sexual relationships. Being aware of your sensuality is another aspect of your sexual being and important to intimacy, or the emotional sharing with a person we care for.

Finally, you may have decided that abstaining from sexual intercourse until marriage is congruent with your value system. Many individuals are choosing sexual abstinence until they enter a committed long-term, monogamous relationship. And while a high percentage of adolescents are reported to engage in sexual intercourse before graduating from high school, there is also a large group of young people committed to sexual abstinence until marriage. If you are choosing to be sexually abstinent, you should know that you are not alone. You will need to decide what it means for you to be abstinent. And abstinence can have different meanings for different people. Finally, even in marriage or other committed relationships, not engaging in sexual activity is sometimes necessary due to illness or other physical conditions. In these situations, it is important to cultivate emotional intimacy and sensuality even though there is no physical intimacy.

Safe Sex

There are at least three methods of physical sexual activity; anal, vaginal, and oral. Anal sex is defined as a sexual act in which a penis is inserted into the anus of a male or female. Although you cannot become pregnant from anal sex, it is a common way to contract sexually transmitted diseases. Vaginal sex is defined as the insertion of the erect penis into the vagina. The use of sex toys and other activities involving the vagina can be considered vaginal sex as well. Finally, the physical act of oral sex is the insertion of an erect penis into another person's mouth or the insertion of someone's tongue into or around a vagina. While you cannot become pregnant from oral sex, you can still contract sexually transmitted diseases. As you can see, all three forms of sex mentioned above open a person up to the risk of contracting a disease. For this reason, engaging in sex should not be taken lightly, at least not without thought and protection.

Protection

If you choose to be sexually active, condoms are the best method to protect yourself from sexually transmitted diseases if they are used correctly and consistently. When used perfectly, condoms are 97–98 percent effective in protecting against most, but not all, sexually transmitted diseases and pregnancy. Always make sure you check the expiration date on the condoms and store them in a dry place away from extreme temperatures. While condoms are an effective form of protection, they are less effective when used improperly. For example, you should avoid oil-based lubricants, such as baby oil or petroleum jelly (Vaseline), when using a condom. Oils react with

THINK ABOUT IT

❏ What influences have shaped your attitudes and values concerning sexuality?

❏ How do you feel about the decision to be sexually abstinent? Can you be abstinent and intimate with someone you care for?

latex and may create small holes that can cause the condom to break. Water-based lubricants, such as K-Y Jelly, are better choices. Additionally, you should never "double wrap" by using two condoms during sex because this can increase the risk of breakage due to the latex of each rubbing against each other. Finally, there is not a male "too big" to wear a condom because a regular-sized condom can stretch to fit over the average person's fist and arm. A large-sized condom can fit over a person's head and shoulders. Size is not an acceptable excuse for not wearing a condom. To become more educated on how to use a condom properly, contact and visit your local student health services or family planning clinic. Many provide free condoms.

As mentioned above, sexually transmitted diseases can also be spread during oral sex. Even during oral sex, a nonspermicidal condom should be worn on the penis to prevent against disease. In addition, there are special condoms solely for use during oral sex. These condoms, known as dental dams, can be used during oral sex to act as a barrier between the vagina or anus and the mouth to protect against disease. If you do not have a dental dam, you can use regular condoms by cutting off the tip, cutting it down the middle, and unfolding it into a rectangle. Regardless of which method you choose, it is important to guard yourself from disease even during oral sex.

Contraception

Contraception is a specific form of birth control that refers to any procedure used to prevent fertilization. Birth control refers to all of the procedures used to prevent pregnancy or conception. Birth control includes all available contraceptive measures, as well as sterilization. Contraceptives vary considerably in their method of use and their rate of success in preventing conception. A few examples of contraceptives are condoms, oral contraceptives, contraceptive patches, the nuva ring, IUDs, spermicides, and diaphragms. The two most common sources of contraception are condoms and oral contraceptive pills. However, no contraceptive is 100 percent effective. There is always a chance of getting pregnant regardless of the kind of contraceptive you choose. The only contraceptive that is 100 percent effective is complete and continuous abstinence.

To prevent unwanted pregnancy, it is important to monitor the woman's menstrual cycle and find a method of birth control that is appropriate for her. Some forms of contraception, such as the pill, must be taken daily. Others, such as the birth control hormone shot, are given every few months. Whatever method you use, it is important to be consistent and follow the directions. It is always a good idea to use condoms in addition to another method of birth control because other contraceptives, such as the pill, will not prevent the transmission of sexually transmitted diseases.

An unplanned pregnancy can be a huge obstacle for any student-athlete. Even during a planned pregnancy many parents have difficult decisions to make and must cope with added stress; however, when a pregnancy is unplanned or unwanted the decisions become even harder. The first decision a woman must make is whether or not to carry the pregnancy to term. Then the mother or parents must decide whether to keep the child, and if so how to raise it and provide for it. Pregnancy and having a child is a permanent life-altering experience. If a female athlete becomes pregnant, this could mean the end of her competitive athletic career, the end of an athletic scholarship, and maybe even a delay or a discontinuation of her college career. Likewise, for a male student-athlete, fathering a child may mean a new set of responsibilities that will affect his future. In general, an unplanned pregnancy can alter student-athletes' athletic dreams, goals, and career path. Ultimately, it could affect everything that they have trained for in their athletic careers, thus student-athletes should be especially careful to make decisions regarding safe sex and contraception.

Sexually Transmitted Diseases (STDs)

Although most students have had a sex education lesson or course during high school, many important facts about sexually transmitted diseases (STDs) and sex may be forgotten or disregarded. Additionally, during sex education classes, students may be too intimidated to ask questions about sex in front of other people, for fear of sounding foolish and because sex can be an uncomfortable topic. When individuals first engage in sexual intercourse and relationships, they typically worry about unwanted pregnancy and focus their concern on birth control. Sexually transmitted diseases are often overlooked. Many forms of birth control do not prevent against STDs. You need to be familiar with various types of sexually transmitted diseases and the precautions needed to prevent transmission. Many people deny that they could ever contract an STD, but the truth is that STDs are very common. In fact, it is estimated that one in three college students have an STD and 1 in 500 college students nationwide have HIV/AIDS.

What do you remember from your high school sex education classes about STDs? Look at Box 9.2; they are common statements about STDs. The correct answers are listed. Can you explain why the statements are true or false?

STUDENT REFLECTION

Box 9.2. How Much Do You Know About STDs?

Do you know why these are true or false?

1. A person with herpes can be completely cured with proper medical treatment.	*False*
2. You can always tell if someone has an STD.	*False*
3. Having a PAP test always includes an STD check.	*False*
4. A person with one sex partner is unlikely to get an STD.	*False*
5. I can get an STD only if I have intercourse.	*False*
6. A consequence of having an STD might be the inability to have children.	*False*

Each year, between 13 and 15 million new cases of STDs are diagnosed in the United States. A quarter of these cases are in young people between the ages of fifteen and nineteen. Many of these individuals are unaware of the dangers posed by STDs or how to prevent or identify them. Most STDs (e.g., gonorrhea, syphilis) can be treated. However, only through abstinence can all STDs be prevented. If not prevented, early diagnosis and treatment can decrease the possibility of serious complications such as infertility in both women and men. Box 9.3 shows a list of common sexually transmitted diseases and facts regarding the symptoms and treatment of STDs.

In addition to the STDs listed in the table, human immunodeficiency virus (HIV) is another major health concern of people who are sexually active. HIV destroys the body's ability to

STUDENT REFLECTION

Box 9.3. What Do You Know About STDs?

Chlamydia
- Chlamydia is curable.
- Up to 80 percent of infected women and up to half of all infected men have no symptoms.

Human Papillomavirus (HPV)
- Human papillomavirus (HPV) infection is a sexually transmitted disease (STD) that can be treated but not cured. However, most infections eventually go away by themselves.
- Most HPV infections cause no serious health problems, but some types of HPV can cause genital warts. Other types sometimes lead to cancer of the cervix, other genital areas, or anus.
- People who use a condom can still get HPV.

Gonorrhea
- Gonorrhea is curable.
- Gonorrhea causes unusual discharge from the vagina, discharge from the penis, pain when you urinate, and abdominal pain in women.

Herpes
- Genital herpes can be treated but not cured.
- People can transmit herpes from the first sign of pain or itching until the scabs fall off.
- People can also transmit herpes some of the time when they have no symptoms.
- People can still get herpes when using condoms.

Syphilis
- Syphilis is curable, but irreversible damage may occur.
- If untreated, syphilis can be very serious, even fatal.

fight off illness, and it leads to AIDS, acquired immune deficiency syndrome, making it the deadliest STD. An estimated 15,000 people contract the HIV virus each day and 33 million people are estimated to be living with HIV or AIDS. In addition, nine out of ten of these people do not even know they are infected. STDs such as syphilis, gonorrhea, and chlamydia actually increase the risk of contracting HIV. The HIV test actually does not detect the presence of the HIV antibodies immediately after risky sexual behavior. HIV usually takes three to six months to show up on a test after the behavior.

Prevention of Sexuality Transmitted Diseases (STDs)

STDs can be prevented though abstinence, a mutually monogamous sexual relationship between uninfected partners, and/or using barrier contraceptives such as condoms. Most barrier contraceptives protect against HIV, gonorrhea, and chlamydia, and provide some protection (but less) against infections that can be transmitted through skin-to-skin contact such as herpes simplex virus, syphilis, and chancroid. While most STDs are curable, there are others that you can have for life.

At the present time hepatitis B virus (HBV) and human papilloma virus (HPV) are the only two sexually transmitted diseases that can be prevented through a vaccination. The hepatitis B vaccination is a series of three shots and is effective only if you receive the vaccine before coming into unprotected sexual contact with someone infected. Recently it has been found that after a person has been exposed to HBV, appropriate treatment given in an appropriate time frame can effectively prevent infection.

Gardasil is the first vaccine developed to prevent cervical cancer and genital warts due to HPV. The vaccine is given in three doses. The vaccine is licensed by the FDA for girls and women ages nine through twenty-six. The vaccine consists of purified, inactive proteins that come from the four most common strands of HPV: types 6 and 11 (which cause 90 percent of genital warts) and types 16 and 18 (which cause 70 percent of cervical cancer). The vaccine does not protect against other types of HPV and does not contain any antibiotics or preservatives. HPV transmission occurs easily with skin-to-skin contact. Condoms may help protect against transmission of HPV but are not fully effective.

Student-athletes are known for taking pride in their physique, fitness, and health, and typically most athletes eat well, exercise, and take care of their bodies. Unfortunately, college students (including student-athletes) do not always take the necessary precautions in protecting their health and bodies from sexually transmitted diseases. Having unprotected sex with someone whose STD status is not known to you is a tremendous risk. Student-athletes who are sexually active can limit their exposure to STDs by using proper protection and limiting partners. Remember that just because you feel healthy and strong does not mean that you are free from STDs because most people are not even aware that they have contracted a disease.

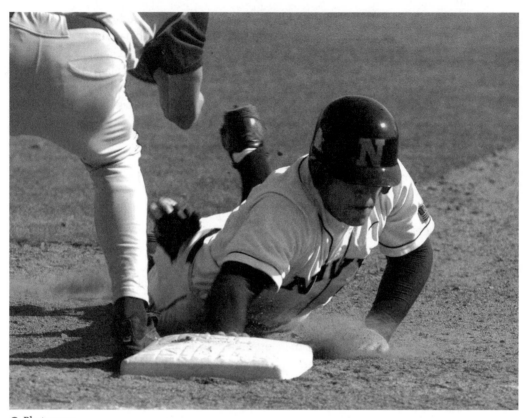

© Photos.com

THINK ABOUT IT

❏ It can be stressful to worry about the correct and most effective contraception that is right for you and your partner. What steps can you take to reduce your fears and get the facts about contraceptives?

❏ For many people, it is difficult to talk openly and honestly about sex. Being sexually responsible involves communication between partners. What do you think partners should know or discuss before having sex?

❏ Describe the differences between males' and females' feelings in regard to sex. Do you think they vary? Do you think it is easier for a male or a female to have sex while in college?

❏ Waiting to have sex can eliminate a lot of pressure and fear. How might you or someone else talk to a partner about developing a closer emotional relationship before a sexual relationship begins?

Sexual Abuse

Rape

Rape is generally considered a crime of sexual aggression in which the victim is forced to have sexual intercourse. It can be vaginal, oral, or anal, and it isn't about sex. Rather, rape is about power and one person exerting control over another. Rape is often described as a violent act that happens to be carried out through sexual contact. Additionally, the issue of consent is important to consider in regard to rape. In the case of rape, consent is not given. Before engaging in sexual activity it is important that both parties give verbal consent and are in a position where they have the capacity to make a decision to give consent or not give consent. As violence in our society increases, the incidence of rape and sexual assault correspondingly rises. Today, there is broader understanding of rape; for example, the term "acquaintance rape" has been coined to refer to forced sexual intercourse between individuals who know each other. The vast majority, about 85 percent, of rapes are acquaintance rapes. Additionally, half of the rapes that happen in colleges are acquaintance rapes that occur during a student's freshman year. Date rape is a specific type of acquaintance rape that involves forced sexual intercourse by a dating partner. On average, 20 percent of college women report having experienced date rape, but a recent report issued by the Bureau of Justice Statistics puts the figure at about 3 percent per year. The difference in these statistics may be due to how people define rape. Rape is typically defined as forced sexual intercourse, but it does not include the numerous sexual assaults that take place each year. In recent years, closer attention has been paid to these sexual crimes, assaults, and acts of sexual victimization. For example, many college students report being kissed and touched against their will, and alcohol is frequently a significant contributing factor in these sexual assault situations. In addition, many incidents of rape and sexual assault on college campuses involve date rape drugs such as GHB and Rohypnol. These drugs are odorless and dissolve in liquids. Often they are slipped into people's drinks and cause a person to become drowsy, disoriented, and uninhibited, and it may even cause amnesia. Alarmingly, even over-the-counter drugs such as eye drops or niacin supplements are being used as tranquilizers to assist in date rape. Finally, there are increased concerns about reported rape targeting gay, lesbian, and transsexual individuals.

As a college student it is important to think about ways you can protect yourself from rape and sexual assault. There are things that you can do to keep yourself safe, such as staying with your friends, going to familiar places, avoiding secluded areas, having a plan of how you will get home, keeping your eye on your drink, and making sure that a friend knows where you are. Likewise, there are myths about date rape that are not true. In Box 9.4 many of the myths are listed. Debunking the myths is important to your safety and protection.

You should also try not to walk alone at night, be aware of your surroundings, and avoid getting into a car if you do not know the driver. Additionally, if you think you are being followed, you

Box 9.4. The Following Are All Myths About Date Rape. What Do You Think About Them?

Date rape is the victim's fault.

She asked for it.

Women "want it."

Gay sex is rough.

Men can't be raped.

When women say "no" they really mean "yes."

Women who dress in sexy clothes want sex.

If a man or woman knows the person, it can't be rape.

People who tease deserve what they get.

A woman can refuse sex if she really wants to.

A real man is sexually forceful.

If a man gets sexually aroused, he needs to have sex.

It's okay to force sex unless the woman or man is a virgin.

If you wanted to have sex, but changed your mind, it is not rape.

A little rough play makes the sex more exciting.

It's not a big deal—it is only sex.

should look for a safe retreat such as a store, fire or police station, or a group of people. Finally, be cautious of first dates, blind dates, or people you meet at a party or bar who push to be alone with you. Most important, trust your instincts and don't put yourself in uncomfortable situations.

Even with precautions, incidents of rape and sexual assault occur. It is important to remember that it is never the fault of the victim and they should not feel guilty. If you or someone you know has been a victim of rape, the information in Box 9.5 will be useful.

Student-athletes have been known to be involved with situations regarding sexual abuse. It is not unusual for teammates to hire strippers, throw wild parties, and be very popular with the opposite sex. Student-athletes are very recognizable on campus and they are often subjected to accusations and rumors, especially regarding their sexual behaviors. As a student-athlete, it is important that you make thoughtful decisions and avoid situations that may lead to sexual misconduct.

Box 9.5. Steps to Take After a Rape Incident

- Call the police immediately to report the assault. The police can take you to the hospital and start gathering information that may help them apprehend the rapist. Fortunately, many police departments now use specially trained officers, many of whom are female, to work closely with rape victims during all stages of the investigation.

- Call a local rape crisis center. These centers are generally operated on a twenty-four-hour hotline basis and they have trained counselors to help victims by contacting the police, escorting them to the hospital, and providing aftercare counseling.

- It is critical that you do not alter any potential evidence related to the rape; for example, don't change your clothes. Additionally, do not take a bath, eat anything, go to the bathroom, smoke, or rearrange the scene of the crime. Instead, wait until all the evidence has been gathered. Evidence stays on your body for seventy-two hours after the incident. Don't worry if you have washed, gone to the bathroom, and changed your clothes; it is still important to go to a hospital and get checked out. The evidence can still be collected up to three days later.

- Report all bruises, cuts, and scratches, even if you think they are insignificant, because these can provide particular information about the attack.

- At the hospital, you will probably be given a thorough pelvic examination; however, you will have to ask for STD and pregnancy tests.

Psychological Issues

Psychologists believe that aside from the physical harm of date rape and sexual assault, a greater amount of emotional damage may occur. Such emotional damage stems from the concept of broken trust, and date rape victims feel particularly violated because the perpetrator was someone they knew and trusted. Once trust is broken, it can be difficult to develop new relationships with other people. Additionally, often there is a double standard in regard to sex in America. For instance, sex typically fuels a man's ego and status with the male population, whereas women who have multiple sexual partners jeopardize their reputation. One way to avoid problems that often stem from sexual encounters is to talk openly with your partner, and find out about your potential partner's sexual history. Unfortunately, even when you are cautious, there is still a chance that your partner desires only a sexual relationship. Any time you have sex with someone, you are allowing yourself to be vulnerable and take the chance of getting hurt. Thus, you should not let your hormones get the best of you. It is important to consider the possible emotional repercussions.

THINK ABOUT IT ✔

- ❑ What behaviors or signs in a relationship might indicate abuse? How can abuse be avoided?
- ❑ How can prior sexual abuse interfere with new relationships? Brainstorm some expectations and steps a couple may need to consider.

In conclusion, student-athletes can experience emotional turmoil that can affect their sports performance. To protect from feeling taken advantage of or from regretting a sexual act, student-athletes should become comfortable with their own sexuality and evaluate what they expect out of relationships and how they feel about sex. By knowing your sexual limits and how you expect to be treated, you are less likely to become a victim of sexual assault. In addition, you may not be inclined to make rash decisions regarding sex and be less likely to feel hurt in relationships.

Team Dynamics

In the Locker Room

Almost everyone has dreaded being naked in front of their peers in a locker room. These moments typically occur during middle school or high school. During adolescence, teens can feel both emotionally and physically naked because they are just becoming comfortable with their changing bodies. They often feel uncomfortable exposing too much of themselves in front of others, especially their peers. For college student-athletes the locker room may still be a place with moments of awkward feelings and discomfort when bodies and sexuality are the topics. At the same time, for college student-athletes it is important to socialize and communicate in the locker room. Often on campus and during competitions student-athletes try not to stand out on their teams and instead they feel a need to bond, fit in, and work for the best interest of the team. Often the locker room becomes a retreat for players, a place for teammates to bond, and/or a place where teammates learn to understand and relate to one another.

During college, however, students (including student-athletes) may be more confident in their bodies but less secure about their sexual identities. For instance, student-athletes who share a common passion for a sport spend huge amounts of time together practicing, competing, and traveling. Some of these athletes share common sexual orientations, but some of their teammates may not. Given these facts, it should not be surprising to find that sexual attractions and relationships occur among student-athletes in sports even though it is not readily accepted or discussed. Thus, locker rooms can be a place for athletes to bond and better understand each other; these moments of team bonding can also be a forum for questions, confusion, hostility, and concern regarding sexuality.

As student-athletes explore their own sexual identity and orientation, there is room for misperceptions and misunderstandings between team members. For example, heterosexuals on a team may have a difficult time accepting and feeling comfortable around a teammate who is gay. Team members may even misunderstand encounters with teammates who are gay, and jump to conclusions that their teammates will make sexual advances. In some instances, heterosexual teammates my feel uneasy about sharing a locker room with teammates who are gay. The uneasiness that they feel is often due to their own insecurities, fear, and curiosity. Regardless, this tension can create a hostile climate in some athletic programs, causing athletes who are gay, lesbian, bisexual, or transsexual to feel threatened, uncomfortable, and even keep their identity hidden in fear of jeopardizing their athletic careers. Contrary to conventional wisdom, a gay/lesbian, bisexual, or transsexual team member who is open about his or her identity is more readily accepted and respected by peers. Additionally, a fellow teammate revealing his or her homosexuality can help heterosexual team members to overcome stereotypes they have about gay athletes. If a team is having trouble being accepting, they must remember that acceptance of an openly gay team member does not require approval of his or her lifestyle. Instead, it requires a respect for difference and a belief that everyone on the team should be safe and treated with dignity and fairness.

The issue of sex does not come up only in the locker room as it relates to identity, orientation, and relationships; it also comes up in conversation. Locker-room discussions often revolve around sex. For instance, female athletes often talk about their relationships with men. Many women's locker room conversations can be edifying or trashy. In fact, females are even more likely than men to talk about sex in critical and detailed ways. The pervasiveness of locker room talk among young women of all backgrounds reflects the feminist movement of the baby boomer generation. Women of the baby boomer era fought to open the doors to bring about free communication among women.

Similar to their socially centered counterparts, male athletes also talk about the opposite sex. Ohio State sociologist Timothy Curry conducted a research study in which he examined men's locker-room conversations. He observed that the men's locker-room discussions were often plagued with bragging, boasting about sexual conquests, and statements that objectified women. Curry discovered that sexually aggressive talk about women usually takes the form of loud, public performance where the male is looking to draw attention. In fact, Curry discovered that if men were going to discuss a woman they were serious about with a teammate, they would discuss it privately in hushed tones away from the group. He also determined that male athletes' "trash talk" escalates as males feel challenged to show their masculinity and prove they are macho. There is a risk that the negative attitudes toward women that are shared by males in the locker room will manifest as sexual harassment and assault. In the most severe cases, this macho bonding results in gang rapes conducted by athletic teams as the ultimate display of their male bonding.

Preventing Sexual Harassment

Scandals involving college student-athletes and reports of sexual misconduct and abuse are highlighted in the news. It is not uncommon for collegiate teams or student-athletes to be accused of sexually assaulting females, harassing homosexuals, making inappropriate comments, or rape. These are just a few examples of incidences where student-athletes have been associated with sexual misconduct. For example, a collegiate football program was discovered hiring adult entertainers to strip and perform lap dances for new recruits to entice them to join the program. Similarly, many players of a collegiate basketball team were suspended because it was discovered that they had hired a prostitute. The members of this basketball team who were involved not only faced serious legal consequences, but also lost their athletic scholarships and the basketball program suffered as a result of their actions. Therefore, as a student-athlete you must realize that your actions can result in serious repercussions. As a

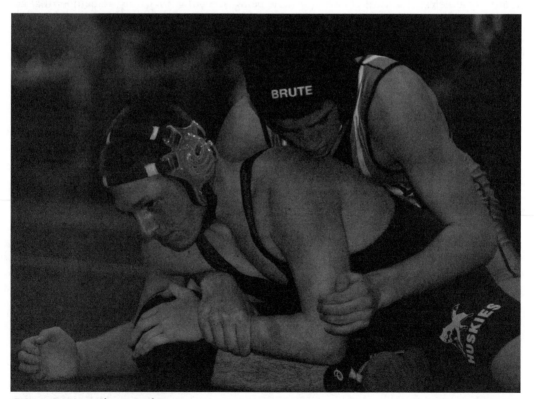

© Larry St. Pierre/ShutterStock, Inc.

collegiate student-athlete, you need to make your teammates feel comfortable and a part of the team. You also need to know how to combat homophobia and create a safe environment for your fellow teammates.

As a student-athlete at the collegiate level, you have the ability to not tolerate sexual harassment behaviors and attitudes that often take place on and off the playing field. As a result of your intolerance or refusal to participate in negative discussions about the opposite sex, gays, lesbians, bisexuals, and transsexuals, you can be an agent of change in the locker room. You also have the power to change stereotypes about homosexuality by creating an environment that is nonthreatening and understanding. It is important for teammates to establish standards for their own conduct regarding sexual behaviors and comments.

It is safe to assume that there are gay, lesbian, bisexual, and transsexual people on your team, and becoming an agent of change simply means not participating in anti-gay behavior or discussions. Instead, you must encourage other teammates to use inclusive language and not assume that everyone is heterosexual. The next step is to talk with administrators about the possibility of offering and/or attending educational sessions regarding homophobia and stereotypes. Furthermore, policies should be established to address homophobic harassment or acts of discrimination when they arise. Finally, promoting an open and tolerant environment is the best thing to do, as well as acknowledging that it is not a special privilege to live without being harassed and discriminated against. In all, if collegiate sports continue to ignore and not address the concerns of gay athletes who feel perverse and ashamed to the point where they become disinterested in playing a sport, they may lose some of their best players in the process.

THINK ABOUT IT

- ❏ Many student-athletes are self-conscious about their sexuality, especially since there is a lot of emphasis placed on sex in sports. Have you ever felt uncomfortable when the topic of sex or sexuality has come up in the locker room? How did you deal with this stress?

- ❏ How would you react to a teammate revealing to you that they were bisexual or gay?

- ❏ How can you be an agent of change in locker-room discussions?

Student-Athletes and Technology

The Internet provides unlimited access to cybersex. As you surf the Internet its pervasiveness is remarkable. Web sites contain everything from amateur fiction, films, and photos to slick triple-X sites. Smut-merchants have staked their claims: from the mainstream and ubiquitous such as Playboy to sites that provide a glimpse into the lives of cruel fetishists.

Cybersex is most commonly performed in Internet chat rooms and on instant messaging systems. The increasing popularity of Webcams has also resulted in an increase in couples using two-way video connections to "expose" themselves to their online chat partners, providing a visual aspect. Chat rooms are the big draw for the cybersexually inclined. The freewheeling conversations range from polite attempts to pornographic chat.

Cybersex differs from phone sex in that it offers a greater degree of anonymity and allows participants to meet partners more easily. In fact, a good deal of cybersex takes place between strangers who have just met online. Wherever you go—and whomever you meet—remember: cybersex is real, at least to some of the people you will meet online.

Engagement in cybersex is not risk free. You simply do not know the individuals with whom you are dealing nor their intent. Students report being harassed, bullied, threatened, and stalked online. Downloading free porn might seem harmless; however, it may cause many computer problems and be a potential source of embarrassment. Furthermore, pornographic materials and images on computer screens, printed, or e-mailed to other people create a hostile and unsafe living and work environment. It is sexual harassment and unacceptable behavior with serious consequences for all parties involved.

Chapter Summary

Almost everyone has sexual experiences at some point in their lifetime, and typically most young adults become sexually active during college. If you are sexually active or planning on being sexually active, you need to take the necessary precautions to protect yourself from sexually transmitted diseases and unintended pregnancy. Additionally, since sex is emotionally driven for many people, you need to share your thoughts and emotions about sex by talking with your partner before having sex. It is wise to discuss previous sexual experiences and what having sex means to you. Discussion and dialogue between partners is important for everyone's safety, health, and emotional well-being. Someone who is not comfortable talking about sex is probably not ready to engage in the act. Furthermore, sexual experiences can sometimes become violent or abusive. Sexual abuse is not limited to rape and assault; rather, it includes derogatory comments and hostile environments as well. You may encounter sexual misconduct in the form of hazing, ridicule of teammates who are gay, and stereotypes of athletes' sexual identity. These attitudes and behaviors are not normal or acceptable and should be reported. Finally, teammates, regardless of their sexual orientation, must be treated with respect and acceptance.

Your Thoughts

1. When do you believe it is acceptable for someone to be in a sexual relationship? Why do you think this varies from individual to individual?

2. How common do you think casual sex is on college campuses? Is this different for student-athletes? What impact do these situations have on students' relationships?

3. STDs are common on college campuses and lead to problems such as infertility and other health hazards. How might you take action and raise awareness to prevent this epidemic?

4. How can you prevent sexual harassment of teammates and other student-athletes? What more can you do to make your school's athletic department free of sexual harassment?

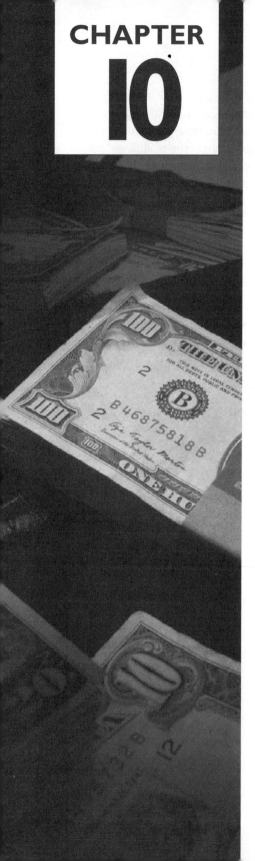

Challenge #8: Gambling and Money

Learning Objectives

After completing this chapter, you will be able to:

- *Recall the NCAA's rules on gambling and consequences for gambling*

- *Identify the different types of gambling that exist on college campuses*

- *Discuss how student-athletes take risks or avoid risks in their daily life*

- *Create a plan for managing your money*

Student-Athletes Say:

- I think gambling on sports is no worse than buying lottery tickets. After all, they both involve taking a chance at winning and playing the odds.

- Every March, I enter a college basketball tournament pool with the guys on my floor. One of my teammates said that I shouldn't do it because it's gambling. What's the big deal? It's only a few dollars.

- For me, gambling makes sporting events more exciting because it gives you a personal investment in the game.

- I am good with money. I spend it as quick as I get it.

- Our team gets together every week for a no-limits poker game. It's just a harmless game, something to do for fun and a great way to bond.

- I am infuriated by the thought that a professional athlete would throw a game because they have money riding on it. I play to win. I think that anyone who places wagers on sports is ruining the competition.

- I'm working part-time plus have school loans. I'll be paying off my school for a long time.

- I talked with someone in the school's athletic department about my money and how I can maybe be a little better at managing it. It's taking me some time to figure it all out.

The rise and popularity of gambling among college students should surprise no one. According to a recent study half of all college men gamble at cards at least once a month. And poker has become a favorite pastime of many college students. In addition, college football and basketball garner so much attention during the school year that many college students (both men and women) participate in friendly bets on their favorite college teams. You can see how gambling has taken root on college campuses across the country.

Gambling, whether it is sports betting or wagering on cards, does not happen just on college campuses. Betting pools for the Super Bowl, NCAA Tournament, and just about any other professional sporting event take place in high schools, colleges, businesses, among friends, in casinos, and online. Gambling has become pretty commonplace in our society. In fact, for many, preparing an NCAA bracket has become a sort of ritual. While one bet a year doesn't mean a person has a problem, placing even small bets may give a person a taste of the world of gambling and may entice them to gamble again. Further complicating the situation is the increase of people using the Internet to place bets and gamble. Many young adults prefer Internet gambling because they have such easy access to it and can remain anonymous.

This chapter is about gambling, but also about money in general. After all, gambling and money go hand in hand. Discussed in this chapter are the NCAA rules prohibiting gambling, money management skills, how to protect your money, and what to do if you have money concerns. As you complete the Student-Athlete Challenge #8: Gambling and Money Self-Assessment in Box 10.1, think about how much attention is focused on sports and gambling. Also think about how you are with money. How are your money-management skills?

Student-athletes are at the nexus of sports betting. On one hand, the NCAA has clear restrictions and consequences regarding student-athletes' involvement with gambling. On the

---

Box 10.1. Student-Athlete Challenge #8: *Gambling and Money Self-Assessment*

Directions: Evaluate each statement on a scale of 1 to 5, from 1 being "never" to 5 being "almost always." For each statement evaluate if your behavior adds value (+), is neutral (0), or decreases value (−) of your student-athlete success in regards to your classes and sport.

Statement	Never			Almost Always		Value Added		
	1	2	3	4	5	+	0	−
1. I gamble at casinos.	❏	❏	❏	❏	❏	❏	❏	❏
2. I play online poker.	❏	❏	❏	❏	❏	❏	❏	❏
3. I talk with my parent or guardian about money	❏	❏	❏	❏	❏	❏	❏	❏
4. I provide inside team information to an outside source.	❏	❏	❏	❏	❏	❏	❏	❏
5. I play poorly to hurt my own team and shave points.	❏	❏	❏	❏	❏	❏	❏	❏
6. I overdraw my bank account.	❏	❏	❏	❏	❏	❏	❏	❏
7. I participate in basketball pools.	❏	❏	❏	❏	❏	❏	❏	❏
8. I play cards for money with friends.	❏	❏	❏	❏	❏	❏	❏	❏
9. I borrow money from my friends.	❏	❏	❏	❏	❏	❏	❏	❏
10. I participate in fantasy sports.	❏	❏	❏	❏	❏	❏	❏	❏
11. I make a budget for each term.	❏	❏	❏	❏	❏	❏	❏	❏
12. I am careful with my money.	❏	❏	❏	❏	❏	❏	❏	❏

other hand, student-athletes are college students who are surrounded and pressured by gambling opportunities that may be legal for other students, but still pose a problem for student-athletes. The story below highlights a gambling situation that a college student-athlete found himself in at one point in his student-athlete career:

> *During my freshman year, my football team had a curfew before games. It was awful! The football team had to stay in while everyone else was out partying and having fun. One night, some players thought it would be fun to play cards. We decided to play for money and everyone was supposed to bring twenty dollars to the table; this way nobody would lose more than twenty dollars.*
>
> *That evening, everything was going fine. People were winning money, losing money, and having a good time. Then, Mike came up with the bright idea of playing Acey Deucey, where two cards are turned up and you bet as much money as you want. If the next card is between the two cards that are shown, you win the pot. However, if you bet and the card is not between the two original cards, then you pay the size of the pot. It sounds fun and exciting, but people started betting more than twenty dollars and the pot got bigger and bigger. At one point, there was three hundred dollars in the pot, and it was my turn. I had a good hand, so I bet it all. I lost the hand and according to the rules, I had to put six hundred dollars in the pot. Unfortunately, I didn't have the money. The guys on the team were furious, and I was embarrassed. One guy got in my face and starting yelling at me, and the captain had to step in and calm him down. Everyone was arguing. It definitely was not the type of team bonding you want to have the night before a big game.*

Gambling takes lots of different forms. It is not just about betting on games or shaving points. It is about money, how you get it, and how you spend the money you have. Your skills of discipline and focus that you developed from playing your sport are particularly important in managing and protecting your money.

Understanding the Odds

Gambling is the act of risking money or valuables in hopes of winning more than you initially risked. People often downplay gambling and see no harm in making a friendly wager or a gentleman's bet. They view gambling as a way to make the game a little more interesting. Gambling is more than just betting money on sports or card games, and it is important to understand that for many individuals gambling becomes a problem in their lives. For some, gambling is simply a social or recreational act. They bet on card games, sporting events, or office pools with their friends and they never risk more than they can afford to lose. For others, gambling begins to cause problems in their lives and consumes much of their time and thoughts. Problem gambling behaviors can often lead to pathological gambling, where a person cannot stop gambling and often loses more money than he or she can afford. Gambling also becomes a problem when it negatively affects other areas of life, such as relationships and health.

Box 10.2. How Much Do Student-Athletes Risk Gambling?

1. How much do you think student-athletes risk harming their athletic and academic careers if they play Internet poker?

   _____ No risk   _____ Great risk

   _____ Slight risk   _____ Moderate risk

2. How much do you think student-athletes risk harming their athletic and academic careers betting on the NCAA basketball tournament?

   _____ No risk   _____ Great risk

   _____ Slight risk   _____ Moderate risk

3. How much do you think student-athletes risk harming their athletic and academic careers if they go to a casino to play the slot machines and card games?

   _____ No risk   _____ Great risk

   _____ Slight risk   _____ Moderate risk

4. How much do you think student-athletes risk harming their athletic and academic careers if they bet on their own games?

   _____ No risk   _____ Great risk

   _____ Slight risk   _____ Moderate risk

5. How much do you think student-athletes risk harming their athletic and academic careers if they purchase lottery tickets?

   _____ No risk   _____ Great risk

   _____ Slight risk   _____ Moderate risk

Source: Adapted from Monitoring the Future, 2007.

Gambling is not limited to monetary stakes placed on games or sporting events; it can also involve taking daily unnecessary chances or engaging in risky behaviors. Every day you take chances and risks and may not even be aware you are gambling. Unnecessary risks are those chances that we take where we know that there is a good possibility for serious consequences and the risk is easily avoidable, but we choose to take it anyway. For example, a player may break

THINK ABOUT IT ✔

❑   How prevalent is gambling on your campus? Within your team? What is your personal stance on gambling?

❑   As a student-athlete, you have little or no time for a part-time job. Do you think it may be very tempting to gamble to make some extra cash, quickly? How else could you deal with financial hardship?

the rules and hope she will not get caught, or a student may choose not to read an assignment for class because the odds the teacher will call on him are low. Whether speeding on the highway and betting that a cop will not catch you or taking a supplement assuming that you will not be given a random drug test, student-athletes take chances and play the odds daily. While you may win in the short term, the long-term consequences of playing the odds can be problematic and place you in a situation where you are risking things that you are unprepared to lose.

Placing Bets

Don't Bet on It

Gambling that involves money occurs more often than you may think. Monetary gambling occurs every time a person takes a risk and bets money when he or she is unsure of an outcome. Typically, people equate gambling with betting on sports or playing cards for money. When student-athletes become involved in gambling, it can mean problems for the student-athletes involved as well as for the universities they represent. Common types of gambling that college student-athletes might participate in include:

- *Sports bets*—Placing bets on sporting events with a bookmaker; for example, horse racing or football. The amount won depends on the probability of that horse or team winning.

- *Betting machines*—Devices such as slot machines or poker arcade games.

- *Casino games*—Variety of card or dice games such as poker, blackjack, or roulette.

- *Bingo*—Board games played by matching assigned numbers that are pulled by a caller.

- *Lottery*—Purchasing a ticket for a random drawing. The winnings depend on how many people play and how many numbers you match.

- *Spread betting*—Bets on the stock exchange and sporting events. Placing bets involves predicting the score or point differentials. Winnings can be large but gamblers have less control over how much they may lose.

Gambling is based on statistics, and those who win at gambling are successful at playing the odds. There is a huge draw for people to gamble. They are driven by the potential of winning big. Unfortunately, what many gamblers do not realize is that the odds of winning are very slim.

If the odds of winning are slim, why are so many people drawn to gambling? Most people are motivated to gamble because of advertisements, the prospect of winning easy money, and the sheer rush that they get from taking a risk. For example, some people see the slogan "You could be the next instant millionaire" and cannot resist the temptation to play. Additionally, some people justify buying lottery tickets because the proceeds from some games actually fund statewide initiatives and benefit schools and senior citizens. But, the truth is that lotteries are an inefficient way to raise money, and only 34 cents from the sale of a $1 ticket fund state programs. The other two-thirds of the sales of lottery tickets go to administrative costs, marketing, and prizes. Additionally, in some states, the odds of winning the jackpot are less that one in thirteen million. With the odds of winning this low, you are better off not playing at all.

Student-athletes may be tempted to play the lottery because many college students have just turned eighteen and are of legal age to buy tickets for the first time. While playing the lottery is legal, it is important for student-athletes to realize that playing the lottery has its risks. Because the odds of winning are slim, playing the lottery is a way that students lose money that they could have been spending on something more important. In addition, taking a gamble on the lottery can entice student-athletes to gamble on other games or events.

Chancing College

Gambling is growing in popularity on college campuses. In the past decade, gambling has become more prevalent, promoted, and organized within colleges and universities. For example, several universities have held poker tournaments on campus, and participation in these school-sponsored events has been high. Furthermore, gambling is becoming more accessible with the new Internet gambling trend. Almost every college student has constant, unlimited access to the Internet and creative ways to generate the funds needed to gamble. Additionally, college campuses are deluged with representatives from credit card companies offering free gifts to students in return for filling out credit card applications. A college student can place wagers over the Internet from their dorm rooms with a credit card and a click of a mouse. A recent survey revealed that 65 percent of undergraduate students have credit cards, and 20 percent have four or more cards. A huge danger of online gambling is that the money spent and lost over the Internet does not feel real. Most students often feel like they are playing with play money. Students place their bets online with a credit card and can quickly accumulate debt without even realizing it.

Student-athletes are confronted with the temptations to gamble, both in sports and on the Internet, but it is important to be aware of the dangers and pitfalls associated with gambling. A study conducted in 1998 by the University of Michigan surveyed 3,000 NCAA male and female student-athletes. Thirty-five percent of student-athletes admitted to placing bets on sports for money while attending college. Alarmingly, over 5 percent of male student-athletes wagered on games in which they participated, provided inside information for gambling purposes, or accepted money for performing poorly in a contest. NCAA investigations have revealed that there is a high incidence of wagering among college students, and it is believed that student bookies are present at every institution.

Losing Big

Even though gambling has become common and in some cases socially acceptable, there are many consequences associated with this activity. Obviously, the biggest danger of gambling is losing. Many college students lose hundreds and even thousands of dollars each year as a result of gambling. This becomes a huge problem for them as it leads to debt and additional financial burdens or stress. In addition to financial consequences, gamblers also experience social consequences that occur when students become more focused on gambling than on other responsibilities such as school, their family, and friends.

Gambling is an addictive behavior, and there are psychological consequences associated with this activity. Some people who begin by gambling socially end up becoming habitual gamblers and even become addicted to it. Someone who has an addiction to gambling has lost self-control regarding the wagers they place. If a person continues to lose, the desire to gamble drives them to try to win their money back. People with a gambling addiction continually raise the stakes and take greater risks. They experience a thrill from taking these risks. Typically, their risks cause them social, financial, and behavioral problems.

Many young people believe they are invincible and in control of their destiny. Many college students (including student-athletes) involved with gambling are willing to risk gambling with their future because they think they have the time to repay their debts. Similarly, student-athletes may be drawn to gambling because they are naturally competitive and they are familiar with taking chances physically in their sports. It may be second nature for them to take chances financially as well. For example, baseball players are taught to make aggressive plays to steal bases and risk that they will be thrown out. Student-athletes who have been trained to take risks for their sport may be more inclined to take chances financially, especially if they believe they will make a lot of money playing professional sports. However, student-athletes must be careful to recognize the consequences involved with gambling. For instance, student-athletes caught gambling, especially on sports, have lost their scholarships, ruined their reputations, and even ended their professional sports careers.

THINK ABOUT IT ✔

❑ Gambling comes in all forms. List ways that student-athletes take chances or gamble daily during practice, competition, and academically. Think about things you do every day.

❑ How can gambling increase stress in a student-athlete's life? How could you help a teammate, friend, or peer with a gambling problem?

❑ Make a list of the positives and negatives about a student-athlete engaging in gambling. Try to think of all of the rewards as well as all of the risks that might result. Which list is longer? Which side would you choose?

Playing the Odds

Gambling with Your Game Plan

Student-athletes have valuable information, and they use it to prepare themselves for competition and to develop a game plan; however, they also can share the information inappropriately for money. A student-athlete can provide spectators and competitors with information such as game plans, players' abilities, players' injuries, and coaching changes that gives these individuals an inside scoop to use to place bets. Sometimes a student-athlete is pressured by friends and family who take advantage of the athlete's knowledge for their own selfish gambling purposes. For instance, they may learn that the point guard for one team is recovering from the flu, and knowing this they may bet against his team. In all, student-athletes should consider the moral and actual consequences for revealing information that they should covet and hold confidential.

NCAA Regulations and Consequences

As the governing body for collegiate athletics in the United States, the NCAA is well aware of the direct threat sports wagering poses to the integrity of each intercollegiate contest. In 1950, the academic community and the public were shocked to learn that the City College of New York men's basketball team was involved in a point-shaving scandal. There have been more recent point-shaving scandals on the campuses of Arizona State University and Northwestern University, and according to federal law enforcement officials, more money was wagered in the

Arizona State case than on any point-shaving scam in the history of intercollegiate athletics. These incidences have been made public by the media, and they have drawn much-needed attention to the problem of sports gambling in intercollegiate sports.

The NCAA has established rules regarding gambling on collegiate sports, and it has also created strict penalties for those who break them. The risks of being caught gambling far outweigh the rewards of gambling on a sporting event. Student-athletes who are caught violating NCAA rules regarding sports wagering jeopardize their athletic scholarships and their eligibility to play, and they may damage their future athletic and career opportunities. A student-athlete's reputation can be completely ruined for being associated with gambling or speculated to have intentionally influenced the outcome of a game. For example, a student-athlete who solicits a bet on any intercollegiate team, takes a bet on any intercollegiate team, accepts a bet on any team representing the institution, or participates in any gambling activity that involves intercollegiate athletics or organized gambling will be banned from playing or competing. The NCAA prohibits participation in any form of legal or illegal sports wagering because of its potential to undermine the integrity of sports contests and jeopardize the welfare of the student-athlete and the intercollegiate athletics community. The NCAA opposes sports wagering because it could potentially place student-athletes in a vulnerable position. But student-athletes are not the only ones that are subject to the NCAA's gambling and sports wagering rules; all coaches, athletic department and conference office staff, as well as all employees of the NCAA must abide by these guidelines or risk facing serious consequences.

The NCAA hopes to educate student-athletes about the dangers of sports wagering and teach them good financial management strategies to deter then from gambling. To do this, the NCAA sponsors sports wagering workshops, anti–sports wagering public service announcements, educational materials, and the "Don't Bet on It" campaign to inform student-athletes about the dangers of sports wagering.

In 2003 the NCAA conducted a study on sports wagering in collegiate athletics. The study surveyed 20,739 athletes, 62 percent males and 38 percent females. The study found that males reported gambling activities, including sports wagering, in a much larger percentage than the females surveyed. Also, student-athletes from Division III were the most likely to gamble and least likely to know the NCAA rules about sports wagering. Data from this study were extrapolated to estimate that more than 66,800 men and 12,500 women were involved in sports wagering in 2003. According to the survey, the top three reasons that student-athletes gambled were for fun, to win money, and for excitement; the top three gambling activities reported were playing cards or board games for money, betting on games of skill (such as darts), and purchasing lottery tickets. The study concluded that student-athletes that gamble and have a potential for problem gambling are more likely to engage in risky or impulsive behaviors, use and abuse substances such as tobacco and alcohol, engage in risky or unsafe sexual behavior, and to have stolen in the past.

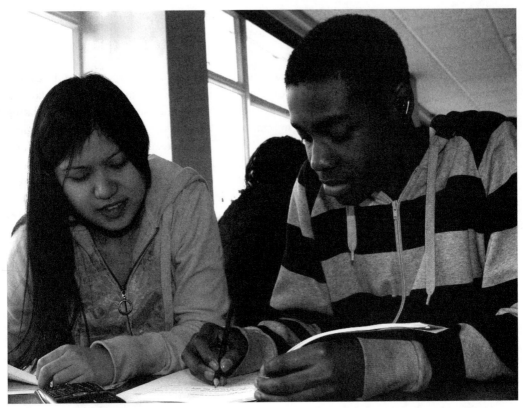

© Laurence Gough/ShutterStock, Inc.

Box 10.3 shows a few questions taken from the 2003 NCAA study focusing on sports wagering as well as the percentage of respondents that answered yes to each question. Read through each question and think about the implications of your answers as they relate to sports wagering in collegiate athletics.

While the vast majority of those who participate in gambling do not experience problems, a small percentage of individuals do experience some problems with gambling. Studies have indicated that approximately 5 percent of the population experience recurrent problems with gambling. On average, it can take eight years to progress from a recreational gambler to a compulsive gambler. Signs of gambling problems include:

- Preoccupation with gambling
- Increasing the size of bets and finding it difficult to quit or cut back while ahead
- Gambling when disappointed or frustrated

- Neglecting one's family, failing at school, or losing a job or a career to gambling

- Selling important possessions to finance gambling

If you have a friend or teammate who you think has a gambling problem, you may be able to help only if the person admits that he or she has a problem. Try to remain supportive and reinforce their efforts toward change while being aware that there may be some steps backward

---

STUDENT REFLECTION

Box 10.3. Questions Taken from the 2003 NCAA National Study on Collegiate Sports Wagering and Associated Behaviors—How Do You Measure Up?

	% of respondents you agree with if you said YES
Do you consider participation in a fantasy league to be "gambling"?	12.9
After you lose money gambling, do you often return another day to try to win back your losses?	14.4
Have you regularly checked the point spreads on games in newspapers or on the Internet?	82.4
Do you place bets on sporting events using a point spread?	9.0
Do you place bets on sporting events by betting on win/loss?	16.0
Do you think sports wagering is okay, as long as you wager on a sport other than the one in which you participate?	59.1
Have you ever placed a sports bet over the Internet?	4.9
Have you ever bet on a college game that involved your team?	2.0
Have you ever bet on a college game that involved another team at your school?	3.6
Have you ever known of a teammate who accepted money or another reward for playing poorly?	1.3
Do you know the NCAA rules on sports wagering?	50.8
Are you aware of any of your coaches or teammates wagering on sports?	13.7

THINK ABOUT IT ✔

- ❏ What would you do if you knew a teammate was involved with point shaving? How would you handle this situation? What are the potential consequences from their actions?
- ❏ Do you think the NCAA rules on gambling are too harsh, just right, or not harsh enough? Explain your answer.
- ❏ How would you react to a family member or friend asking you for inside information about your team?
- ❏ As technology advances, what potential problems do you foresee regarding the multimillion-dollar business of sports gambling?

as a normal part of the recovery process. You can also encourage the person to make contact with organizations like the campus counseling and mental health center, Gamblers Anonymous, or your state's Council on Problem Gambling. Finally, to help your friend or teammate you can schedule activities that are not related to gambling, as well as curb your own gambling behaviors, and educate yourself about problem and compulsive gambling.

Your Money

One attraction of gambling is the money. People are lured by the fantasy of making money the easy, quick, and fun way. You are working at everything else in your life, so why not relax and get some extra easy money? You may also need the money and feel pressured to be involved with gambling (and/or feel pressure from your friends to be part of the "fun"). Helpful to many student-athletes when feeling money pressure is to step back and try to figure out the money in their lives, and how to manage it and make good use of what they have. Also helpful is getting some help dealing with money concerns they have.

Managing Your Money

Most college students are worried about paying tuition bills. Tuition and fees vary widely depending on the school. In general, in-state tuition is cheaper than out-of-state, and public school tuition is less than private school tuition. Don't forget that tuition and fees are only one part of the cost of attending college. Books and supplies have to be considered. Whether you live on or off campus, there will be cost-of-living expenses for housing, food, and transportation. And there are always miscellaneous expenses for personal items and entertainment. For an average college student at a four-year public university, total college costs after four years will amount to about $69,112. And unless you or your parents planned and saved, a good part of that is going to be debt.

But as you look at your classmates, you can assume that financial situations differ depending on life situations. Some students have athletic scholarships that enable them to go to school for no cost to them or their family, while other students' parents and families may be paying all or most of the bill. Many students will have to repay loans after they have completed their educational experience. Still, many students work at least part-time to pay bills and have spending money for the things that they want to buy. One of the most common bad spending habits is not being able to understand clearly the difference between needs and wants.

A necessity is something that you would find it difficult or uncomfortable to live without such as food, clothing, and shelter. While wanting a few luxuries in life is not necessarily entirely bad and can motivate you to accomplish goals, having too many wants can be dangerous and sneak up on you when you least expect it.

College is a time for you to learn money management skills because it is the first time you will be handling money without parental or guardian supervision. Whether your family will be supporting you financially or you choose to get a part-time job, it is crucial for you to learn how to budget now so you will have proper money management skills in the future. The basics of budgeting are the same for student-athletes as they are for anybody else: The first step in developing a college budget is becoming familiar with the necessary expenses or costs of living. These costs can be broken down into two categories: fixed and variable. Fixed costs can include tuition, rent/room and board, car payments, car insurance, and parking fees. These costs are set figures. Variable costs can include entertainment, gasoline, food, utilities, hygiene necessities, clothes, car maintenance, books, cell phone bills, and/or club dues. These costs can vary from month to month.

After you become familiar with your fixed and variable costs, you will need to determine if your sources of income will cover the costs (Box 10.4). Income can include the money from a part-time job, allowance from home, grants, scholarships, or loans. If your expenses are less than your income, you're in good shape as long as you stick to your spending plan. If your expenses are more than your income, you need to find ways to cut spending or increase your income. For example, to help reduce expenses, you may be able to carpool with friends if you commute to campus or limit entertainment to once a week. To help increase income, you may be able to get a part-time job if you don't already have one. Just remember that your schoolwork comes first.

After completing the budget worksheet in Box 10.4, and as time goes on and you start spending money, you may realize that your original budget needs to be revamped. You may find out that you need more money or that you have way too much money to waste. Either way, you will need to make appropriate adjustments to the budget.

REFLECTION

STUDENT REFLECTION

Box 10.4. What Is Your Student College Budget?

Projected Income for Semester		*Estimated Expenses for Semester*	
Parental contributions	$	Tuition and fees	$
Savings contributions	$	Books/supplies	$
Work/study during term	$	Rent/housing	$
Other work during term	$	Board/meals	$
Scholarships	$	Phone/utilities	$
Grants	$	Clothing	$
Loans	$	Laundry	$
Public benefits	$	Personal expenses	$
Social Security, etc.	$	Recreation	$
Other income	$	Child care	$
		Medical/dental	$
		Credit card debt	$
		Savings	$
		Computer	$
		Transportation (gas, auto, bus)	
		Other expenditures (e.g., postage, pocket money)	$
Total semester income	$	Total semester expenses	$

Protecting Your Money

As a student-athlete you are familiar with the concept of protecting a lead. Your team is ahead. It is late in the game. You need to keep to your plan and at the same time be disciplined and focused. Likewise, you need to be disciplined and wise in your money management. There are a number of actions you can take to protect your money.

Bank in your college community. Open an account with a bank with an office on campus or within walking distance of campus. Ideally, the same bank will have an office close to your parents' or guardians' home, too, so if need be, your parent or guardian can access it (with your permission). Look for banks that offer checking accounts with no minimum balances and/or monthly fees and a savings account that can be used as overdraft protection for the checking.

Savings and checking accounts. Go to the bank and open checking and savings accounts to access your money. A savings account will allow you to save money. A checking account will help you spend money. You can get money from your checking account by writing checks. Debit, check, or ATM cards can also be used to get money from your checking account. Make sure to keep track of your spending and balance by writing it down somewhere like the checkbook check register. Finally, try to keep some money in your savings account in case of an emergency.

Cash and debit card vs. checks. Make sure to carry some cash on you at all times. Using cash to buy things is easy. Debit, check, and ATM cards draw money directly from your account. Banks often let you draw money out of your account even if you do not have enough money, but then they charge you a fee for overdrawing your account. Be careful. Also, when you receive a check either from work or as a gift and you deposit it in your account, give the check a few days to post before trying to withdraw those funds. Checks take time to clear, so you may not be able to access the money as quickly as you like.

Other people making deposits in your account. If you are worried about your spending, you can keep a joint account with your parents or another adult that you trust. They can monitor your spending and help you stay on track. They can also deposit money into the account if you are running a little short on cash. Some banks offer this service on the Internet. That way, if you live far away from your family, you can still have shared bank accounts.

Protect information. Do not use your address, phone number, birth date, or team number as your pin number. Guard your debit, ATM, check card, and credit card PIN numbers. On your debit, ATM, check cards, and credit cards write the words "picture ID required" under the signature area on the back. Be careful of e-mails with fake bank Web links trying to trick you to give them your account information. Make sure to destroy all papers and receipts that have any account information before throwing them away.

Avoid Internet banks. Do not use banks that are solely on the Internet. Some banks offer on-line features and this is safer. If you must or already use an Internet bank, make sure it is legitimate and that your deposits are federally insured. One way to verify the legitimacy of the bank is to visit the "About Us" section on the bank's Web site, where you may find a brief history of the bank, the official name, and the address of the bank's headquarters. The major concern with Internet banks is that the Internet is supposed to make things faster; however, you might have to wait a long time for checks to clear and to get access to your money. Also, if there is a problem you need to depend on their customer service telephone lines, which can take a lot of time and be frustrating to use. Finally, deposits to an Internet bank account can be slow. If you get a check, such as a student loan check, and you want to start earning interest, you can expect to wait.

Credit cards. Do not be fooled by short-term zero-interest offers that balloon to 21 percent or higher. You pay twice for all items that you want to buy on credit: once for the item you buy and again on the interest when you do not pay for the item at the end of the month when the bill is due. Never sign up for a credit card unless you are capable of paying the total balance on time at the end of every month.

Financial Concerns

Knowing how much money you have at any one time is a concern for many college students (including student-athletes). You are busy. And your money is tight. And there are so many ways you can spend your money. To get some control over your spending, get in the habit of checking your monthly bank statements. Each month your bank will mail you a paper statement of your account information and summary. Banks also offer online banking with the benefit to reconcile your checking account online. Some people like online statements because you don't have to worry about lost or stolen mail and you can usually access each month's statement earlier than the paper statement would arrive. Try to review and balance your account using the monthly statements.

If you think there is a problem, talk with your bank or creditors sooner rather than later. When you put financial problems on the back burner, the debt will only get larger and more difficult to resolve. As soon as you begin to experience trouble, contact your bank or creditors to inform them that it may be difficult for you to make payments. Most banks and creditors will assist you with developing a repayment plan. Banks and creditors do not want to lose your business. If the bank or creditors have turned the problem over to a collection agency, it is too late and it is time to talk with someone you trust such as parents, relatives, or financial counselors to help you deal with the collectors.

Also, notify your bank or credit card company immediately if you lose your credit card or debit card or suspect fraudulent activity on your account. These institutions will be able to put a hold on your account so that a thief cannot use the card and spend all your money. In addition, certain credit card companies and banks offer additional card protection plans so that you are not liable for any transactions that others may make on your account. You may wish to look into these sorts of plans to better protect your accounts from theft. Overall, the best way to protect your finances is to keep your information private, review your account statements, save receipts, and monitor your accounts regularly.

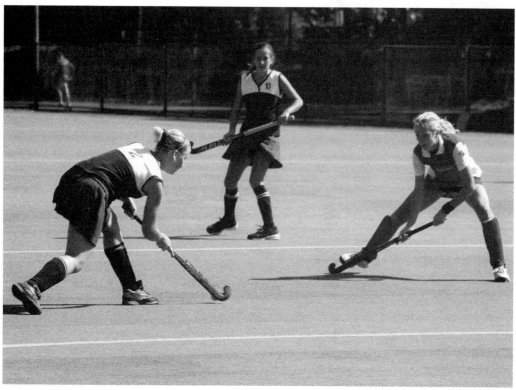

© Alexander Kalina/ShutterStock, Inc.

Overall, if you want to be financially independent, remember these simple do's and don'ts:

- Do not spend more than you have.
- Do always pay your credit card bill in full each month.
- Do not buy on impulse.
- Do buy sale items and shop discount stores.
- Do have your paycheck directly deposited.
- Do start a savings plan.
- Do pay by check, debit card, or credit card to keep track of purchases.
- Do create a semester-by-semester budget.

THINK ABOUT IT

- Why is money management important for college students?
- It is easy to lose track of how much money you have at any given time. What are some things you can do to keep track of your spending?
- What advice would you give to a teammate who is managing his or her own money for the first time?

PLUGGED IN TO SPORTS

Student-Athletes and Technology

With the growing number of computer security issues, it's crucial for college students to know how to be protected from potential threats. There are a few things you should know so that your computer is not the victim of harmful pranks, malicious attacks, and other incidents that might happen during college. All laptop and tablet computer owners should be aware that their computers are at a greater risk of theft, so never leave laptops unattended. You can also buy a locking cable; they are cheap, portable, lightweight, and strong. Make sure to put identification on the laptop itself such as your phone or e-mail address on an engraved identification tag and record your laptop's serial number and network hardware address to track it.

To protect your computer from viruses, never open e-mail attachments from unknown sources, and use antivirus software and keep it updated. Schools usually require computers on their network to have antivirus software in order to connect to the Internet or any other resource on the network. Visit your school's technology help desk to obtain the software. Most schools offer the software to their students free of charge. Also, make sure to scan for adware and spyware programs to protect against applications that get installed on your machine without your permission. Similarly, install and run a personal firewall to block unwanted Internet access through your computer. Finally, if you are using a computer in the lab on campus, press Windows + L to bring your computer to the password-protected screen when you leave it and want to come back. If you are using a Mac computer, press Shift, Command, Option, Q to bring the computer to the password-protected screen. Your network account and password act as your identity on your college's network. To help ensure that no one else besides you can access your e-mail or other files, do not give out your password to anyone.

Chapter Summary

The number of college students who participate in various forms of gambling has risen in recent years. This is due, in part, to increased publicity of sports and sports wagering and an increase in access to gambling on Internet sites. As a student-athlete, you are surrounded by the realm of sports betting and every player knows the temptation to bet. The urge to take risks and gamble is completely normal, but when it gets out of control it can turn destructive. Risky gambling behavior can lead to problems at school, at work, in your personal relationships, and in the overall quality of your life. It can make you feel as though you are at the mercy of unpredictable and powerful emotions. Gambling can lead to financial troubles and debt in addition to psychological and social consequences.

Money and financial troubles are common stressors for college students, and gambling only makes these worries worse. Students, particularly student-athletes, have busy schedules and usually do not have time to work and earn enough money to live on. Many students rely on savings, help from family or friends, and student loans to make ends meet. Students should use college as an opportunity to learn how to manage their money, live within the framework of a budget, and build credit. The financial decisions you make early on will set a foundation for how you manage your money in the future.

Your Thoughts

1. Your roommate is online gambling every night for hours; his credit card debit is increasing and you suspect that he is stealing. How should you approach your roommate? What steps might you take to help him?

2. Think of a time when you "gambled" in a game, match, or competition. Likewise, maybe there is a specific incident when you went against your coach's instructions or took a risk during competition. Describe that situation and the outcome of your decision to chance it.

3. If you were on the NCAA committee creating the rules and consequences for student-athletes regarding gambling, what rules would you add, revise, or remove?

4. Who knows the most about your financial status? Do you have one person who you trust to discuss your current financial status and money management skills? What can you do to improve how you use and manage your money?

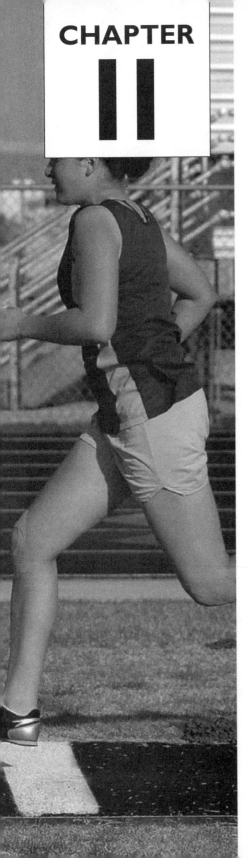

CHAPTER 11

Addressing the Challenges: Resources, Help, and Support

Learning Objectives

After completing this chapter, you will be able to:

- *Identify resources on campus and in the community that student-athletes can utilize for help in facing challenges*

- *Understand that student-athletes do not have to face these challenges alone*

- *Ask for help!*

- *Build support*

Student-Athletes Say:

- I couldn't win without my teammates, my coach, family, and friends. They give me so much.

- Sometimes the stress and anxiety to perform well on the field and in the classroom can be overwhelming and I find it difficult to ask my parents for help when dealing with the stress.

- One day at practice, I had difficulty learning the play and I had to ask the coach to show me the move over and over. I did not want to ask this in front of my teammates, but I had to learn it.

- My parents thought that they could help me get rid of my depression by loving me more. I eventually had to seek out the professional help that I needed.

- I did not want to ask the trainer for help with an injury. I tried to hide the injury because I did not want to go back to physical therapy, but my coach eventually noticed.

- As the star of my baseball team in high school, I thought that my swing was perfect. But in college, I came to realize that I needed help so I could be more consistent and hit the ball farther.

- My math class is really difficult and I'm afraid of looking stupid if I ask my teammate who is in the same class to work with me and figure it out.

- I had a rough season and didn't get as much playing time as I expected. I didn't know if I even wanted to try out for the team again next year. I felt that I needed some advice and support, so I asked a friend to help me analyze the situation. With my friend's support, it was much easier for me to reach a decision.

This book is about you as a student-athlete succeeding at college in your classes and on the playing field. It addresses your needs and anxieties and supports you in your college experience. The college years are times of achievement and success as well as much anxiety and soul searching. As a competent and caring individual, you make good health decisions and health choices in pursuing your student-athlete dreams.

Addressing the eight challenges discussed in this book requires you to take action. Each one of the challenges is already in your life and the lives of your friends and teammates. At whatever your level of involvement and whether the challenges are positives (+'s) or negatives (−'s) in your life as a college student-athlete, these are constants in your life. Given this reality, what are the actions you need to take to be a successful college student-athlete? There are three actions:

1. Find resources

2. Ask for help

3. Build support

While these actions cannot guarantee success in classes and athletics, they can get you pretty far down the road of success.

Find Resources

An important part of the college environment is the services provided to students. Most universities provide students with lots of activities and services to address learning, religious, recreational, emotional, social, and physical health needs. These resources are in addition to those of the athletic department, which typically has its own support services for athletes that include medical services, tutoring, mentoring, and recreational, family, and community activities.

Knowing how to ask for help is critical. It is equally important to know how and where to look for help, or in other words, how to get help. In an emergency you can always call the campus police or public safety office, but for the challenges that student-athletes face it is almost never that clear where to find help. You need to do some investigation.

It is probably the easiest to explore this idea by thinking, what if you, a teammate, or friend had a concern? Where would you turn? Where might you go for help? One answer to that question is to find a place on campus that might be a support. How well do you know the services available to you on campus? Below is a list of campus services that probably operate on your campus. See how many you can locate (careful—the names may be slightly different). When you find them, consider writing down the locations and maybe the Web sites where you can find out more about their services and activities. There is space in Box 11.1 to write additional services unique to your campus.

Once you have found a service or activity that seems like it may suit you, it's time to call or check its Web site to learn more. Think about what you might want to know. It sounds simple, but before calling, make sure you know what you need help with and what kind of help you need. This will make it easier for everyone involved. Provide as much detail as you can. To start,

STUDENT REFLECTION
STUDENT REFLECTION

Box 11.1. Campus Resources for the Student-Athlete

University Counseling Center	Student-Athlete Academic Services Center
Disability Resources and Services	Dean of Students
Health Education Center	Residence Life
Health Services	Student Affairs
Employment, Job, and Career Services	Intramural and Recreational Sports
Student Clubs	Sexual Assault Services
University Chaplaincy (Clergy)	International Student Services
Public Safety (Police)	Diversity and Cultural Services

it may be easiest to ask about hours, activities, costs, and staff who work with students. The person who answers the telephone may be able to answer the bulk of your questions. The Web site may also have most of the information.

You should know that almost all of the services provided on campus (especially those related to health, learning, and personal challenges) are confidential. The person you are talking with at the service will not share or disclose your information to anyone (including parents and coaches) without your permission. In fact, to reinforce and support your privacy, colleges and universities link their athlete support programs with the school counseling services to ensure privacy and confidentiality.

THINK ABOUT IT ✓

❏ Take a walk. Pick one of the campus resources, get its exact location, and make a visit to "check it out." Stop in and ask to talk to someone to get more information about its services.

❏ Are there services off campus you know of that might be worthwhile for you and your teammates to know about? Get information (address, telephone numbers, service hours, Web site) to share.

❏ Talk with your friends who attend other colleges. Are there resources and services that you have heard about from them on their campuses that you would like to have available on your campus?

Ask for Help

Going to others for help is something we're supposed to learn early on. Maybe we do, but all too often, as we get older and more self-reliant (which is obviously a good thing) we tend to forget that everyone could use a little help now and then. According to researchers, student-athletes are often reluctant to seek help for two reasons.

- Student-athletes have tight schedules. Often they do not have much flexibility, and they may worry that spending time getting help to address a concern may take time away from priority activities such as practice and study. They may postpone asking for help, hoping for improvement or a solution.

- Student-athletes worry about being judged. Many student-athletes may view asking for help as a sign of weakness or believe that something is really wrong with them. You need to know that it is pretty common to feel awkward or embarrassed when you can't figure something out; just remember it happens to everyone and there are times when the smart thing to do is to get help.

As a student-athlete you are a disciplined, hard-working, focused individual who usually does not need much help with things—or at least that's how it seems. You are a self-starter and a self-motivator who can learn and do anything. The truth is that there are many times when we can all use or need help. Everyone gets stressed out and feels in over their heads once in a while, and it's no big deal to call out for a little help now and then. In fact, asking for help when it's needed can make your life easier. One of the hardest things is to know when you need help. Many student-athletes think they can do it all, which often leads to frustration or worse. It is worse to not act: something may get broken or you might be pushed into a situation beyond easy repair by trying to go it alone. When you start to get stuck, think about your problem, and if you can use help, ask. Talk to someone you trust about how he or she might ask for help with a concern; knowing how this person would handle such a situation might make it easier for you. If you're unsure, think about the consequences of not asking for help. Finally, try not to wait until it's too late. Try to ask for help as soon as you think you might need it.

How do you ask for help? Each person has his or her own unique style. However, asking for help involves sharing your situation, feelings, and thoughts as honestly as possible with another person to let them understand what is going on. You let other people get involved in helping you decide what it is that you want to do. You still need to be and are responsible for deciding what to do. For example, you might ask, "Would there be a good time for you to show me how you did that on the course Web site? I would really appreciate it," or "Could we get together some time in the next couple of days to talk about the assignment?"

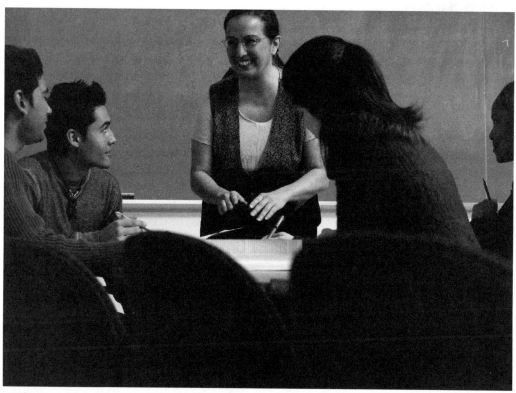

© Photos.com

Sometimes you can state the need you have and try to get someone else involved. For example, you might say, "The meeting is a week away and it's apparent that I won't be able to complete this assignment by myself. Would you be willing to find time in the next two evenings to work on this with me?"

What if you get a "no" when you ask? Perhaps that individual is drowning in work as well. How about going out on a limb and asking if you can help them? Sure, you still have to find some help for yourself, but by helping this person, you may be building a relationship so that they drop everything the next time to help you.

Finally, by getting in the practice of asking for help you develop a network of people who you can ask for help. Likewise, they can ask you. When this happens, asking for help changes from being thought of as a sign of weakness to being thought of as a sign of trust and honesty among friends, which builds relationships, increases your morale, and makes you feel like you're not alone and that you're part of the group, part of the team.

Build Support

Sharing the resources you find on and off campus and asking and giving help with friends builds a network of support for you. Your network of support acts as a buffer against the ups and downs of dealing with the challenges of being a college student-athlete. There is nothing better than being able to call a family member or friend to share a frustration or sad moment as well as achievement and success. You just feel better.

Cultivating social support can take some effort. Here's how to develop and maintain strong and healthy social ties: First, social support is a network of family, friends, colleagues, and other acquaintances you can turn to, whether in times of crisis or simply for fun and entertainment. Just talking with a friend over a cup of coffee, visiting with a relative, or attending a church outing is good for your overall health. Your friends and social contacts may encourage you to change unhealthy lifestyle habits, such as excessive drinking, or they may urge you to visit your doctor when you feel depressed, which can prevent problems from escalating.

THINK ABOUT IT ✔

- ❏ What is your style in asking for help? How do you prepare to ask for help?
- ❏ Have your requests for help been turned down? Have you asked for help and been told no? What happened?

Social support can also increase your sense of belonging, purpose, and self-worth, promoting positive mental health. It can help you get through a divorce, a job loss, the death of a loved one, or the addition of a child to your family.

And you don't necessarily actually have to lean on family and friends for support to reap the benefits of those connections. Just knowing that they're there for you can help you avoid unhealthy reactions to stressful situations.

Some people benefit from large and diverse social support systems, while others prefer a smaller circle of friends and acquaintances. In either case, it helps to have plenty of friends to turn to. That way, someone is always available when you need them, without putting undue demands on any one person. You don't want to wear out your friends.

Developing and maintaining healthy social ties involves give and take. Sometimes you're the one giving support and other times you're on the receiving end. Recognize who is able to provide you with the most support. Letting family and friends know you love and appreciate them will help ensure that their support remains strong when times are rough.

Your social support system will help you if you take time to nurture friendships and family relationships. Here are some things to keep in mind:

- Accept invitations to events, even if it feels awkward and difficult at first.

- Don't wait to be invited somewhere. Take the initiative and call someone.

- Set aside past differences and approach your relationships with a clean slate.

- Take part in campus and community organizations, residence hall or campus events, or family get-togethers.

- Strike up a conversation with the person next to you in class or at a local gathering. You could be introducing yourself to a new friend.

- Talk about things that interest other people. Be an alert listener.

- If you live in the residence halls, take advantage of group activities to meet people and be physically active, such as participating on an intramural activity team.

- Find people who also have an interest in developing healthy lifestyle behaviors and get involved in activities with them.

Some of the people you routinely interact with may be more demanding or harmful than supportive. Give yourself the flexibility to limit your interaction with those people to protect your own psychological well-being. Social support provides a sense of belonging, security, and a welcoming forum in which to share your concerns and needs. And you may get just as much out of friendships and social networks where you're the source of comfort and companionship, too.

Relationships change as you age, but it's never too late to build friendships or choose to become involved. The investment in social support will pay off in better health and a brighter outlook for years to come.

THINK ABOUT IT

☐ Teammates, coaches, professors, friends, and family members can all be sources of social support. Who is in your network of support? Give some examples of support you have received and given during the current school year.

☐ How do you build your social support? How can you expand and increase your support?

PLUGGED IN TO SPORTS

Student-Athletes and Technology

These days, technology can make it easier to keep in touch with family members and friends. For example, your family can get in touch any time of the day by using an e-mail list to spread news or swap helpful resources. A group Web site can also be a place where your friends and family can share digital files, such as photos. You can also all get together on the Web site for scheduled chats. To get started, check out some of the popular online group services, such as Yahoo! Groups (groups.yahoo.com), MSN Groups (groups.msn.com), AOL Groups (groups.aol.com), or Friendster (friendster.com). Families can also use Blip TV (blip.tv) to upload home videos for free, and you can use sites such as YouTube (youtube.com) to edit video. Similarly, many people are choosing to send greeting cards or e-cards for special occasions such as birthdays, anniversaries, and so on. Finally, using a video conferencing service or Internet phone service like Skype, you and your partner, friend, or relative can not only talk with one another, but also see each other's facial expressions. Overall, the Internet can allow you to maintain a connection with your hometown friends, family, and culture, even when those people and interests may be thousands of miles away from you.

Chapter Summary

Facing the student-athlete challenges takes action. The actions discussed in this chapter (finding resources, asking for help, and building social networks) help you succeed as a college student-athlete. The challenges are real. Over your college career and beyond the challenges do change, but by knowing where to turn, asking for help, and building support you will be in charge of your life: making the choices and decisions you want to make, playing and working on achieving your goals both in the classroom and on the playing field.

Your Thoughts

1. Think of asking and getting help as treating yourself well. You work hard and desire the support and attention. How do you treat yourself well, even when you are feeling bad?

2. Every school term and season ends. How do you, family, and friends remember and celebrate your accomplishments of a particular term and season? How do you share and preserve the memories?

3. You will always be a college student-athlete even after you graduate from college. How do you stay connected with teammates who graduated and completed their college sports eligibility? How will you stay connected with your teammates and coaches (and professors, too) when you are done playing sports in college?

References

Chapter 1

Hopkins, G. (2005). *Athletes need to make the grade.* Retrieved May 8, 2006, from http://www. education-world. com/a_lesson/newsforyou/newsforyou004.shtml.

Johnson, D. (2003). *Reaching out: Interpersonal effectiveness and self-actualization* (8th ed.). Boston: Person Education, Inc.

National Collegiate Athletic Association. (2007). *Compliance.* Retrieved November 9, 2007, from http://www. ncaa.org.

National Collegiate Athletic Association. (2007). *Rules and bylaws.* Retrieved November 9, 2007, from http://www. ncaa.org.

Special Olympics. (2005). *Coaching guides.* Retrieved May 8, 2006, from http://www.special olympics.org/Special+Olympics+Public+Website/English/Coach/Coaching_Guides/Aquatics/ Aquatics+Rules+Protocol+and+Etiquette/Sportsmanship.htm.

Chapter 2

Davis, M., Robbins-Eshelman, E., & McKay, M. (2000). *The relaxation and stress reduction workbook* (5th ed.). New York: MJF Books.

Donatelle, R. J. (2003). *Access to health* (8th ed.). San Francisco, CA: Benjamin Cummings.

Ellis, A., & Harper, R. A. (1961). *A guide to rational living.* Chatsworth, CA: Wilshire Book Co.

Ellis, A., & Harper, R. A. (1997). *A guide to rational living* (3rd ed.). Chatsworth, CA: Wilshire Book Co.

Hahn, D. B., Payne, W. A., & Mauer, E. B. (2004). *Focus on health* (7th ed.). New York: McGraw-Hill.

McKay, M., Davis, M., & Fanning, P. (1997). *Thoughts and feelings: Taking control of your moods and your life* (2nd ed.). Oakland, CA: New Harbinger Publications.

Payne, W. A., Hahn, D. B., & Mauer, E. B. (2005). *Understanding your health* (8th ed.). New York: McGraw-Hill.

Seaward, B. L. (2005). *Managing stress: Principles and strategies for health and wellbeing* (5th ed.). Sudbury, MA: Jones and Bartlett.

Towbes, L., & Cohen, L. (1996). Chronic stress in the lives of prospective predictions of distress. *Journal of Youth and Adolescence, 25*(2).

Chapter 3

Ferrett, S. (2006). *Peak performance: Success in college and beyond.* Boston: McGraw-Hill.

Gardner, H. (1993). *Multiple intelligences: The theory in practice.* New York: Basic Books.

Gardner, H. (1999). *Frames of mind: The theory of multiple intelligences.* New York: Basic Books.

Langan, J. (2003). *Ten skills you really need to succeed in college.* Boston: McGraw-Hill.

Nist, S., & Holschuh, J. (2006). *College success strategies.* New York: Penguin Academics.

Chapter 4

Adirim, T. A., & Cheng, T. L. (2003). Overview of injuries in the young athlete. *Sports Medicine, 33,* 75–81.

American Pain Foundation. (2007). *Pain notebook.* Retrieved November 9, 2007, from http://www.painfoundation.org/Publications/Notebook.pdf.

American Pain Foundation. (2007). *Pain resource guide: Getting the help you need.* Retrieved November 9, 2007, from American Pain Foundation. (n.d.) *Pain notebook.* Retrieved November 9, 2007, from http://www.painfoundation.org/Publications/Notebook.pdf.

Clarkson, M. (1999). *Competitive fire: Insights to developing the warrior mentality of sports champions.* Champaign, IL: Human Kinetics.

Competitive Edge. (2006). *Rebounding from injuries: The mental side of athletic injuries: A coach's and athlete's guide to psychologically rebounding from injury.* Retrieved April 27, 2006, from http://www.competitivedge.com/resources_rebounding_from_injuries.htm.

Fritts, R. *Coping with loss: Depression and acceptance.* Retrieved April 27, 2006, from http://www.cedarlane.org/ooserms/s000227.html

Granito, V. J. (1997). Athletic injury experience: A qualitative focus group approach. *Journal of Sport Behavior, 24.*

Hackney, R. G. (1994). ABCs of sports medicine: Nature, prevention, and management of injury in sport. *British Medical Journal, 308,* 1356–1359.

Heil, J. (1993). *Psychology of sport injury.* Champaign, IL: Human Kinetics.

Krames, E. (2007). *My treatment: Pain medicine: Using the tools of the trade.* Retrieved November 9, 2007, from the National Pain Foundation Web site: http://www.nationalpain foundation.org/mytreatment/.

Levinthal, C. F. (2002). *Drugs, behavior and modern society.* Boston: Allyn & Bacon.

Nemeth, R. L., von Baeyer, C. L., & Rocha, E. M. (2005). Young gymnasts' understanding of sport-related pain: A contribution to prevention injury. *Child: Care, Health & Development, 31,* 615–625.

Orchard, J. M., & Best, T. M. (2002). The management of muscle strain injuries: An early return versus the risk of recurrence. *Sports Medicine, 12,* 3–5.

SpineUniverse.com. (2007). *Questions you should ask about pain and pain treatment.* Retrieved November 9, 2007, from http://www.spineuniverse.com/displayarticle.php/article1613.html.

Taylor, J., & Taylor, S. (1998). Pain education and management in rehabilitation from sports injury. *Sport Psychologist, 12,* 68–88.

Chapter 5

Boyle, M. A., & Anderson, S. L. (2004). *Personal nutrition.* Belmont, CA: Thomson Wadsworth.

Connor, B. O., Fasting, K., Dahm, D., & Wells, C. (2001). *Complete conditioning for the female athlete: A guide for coaches and athletes.* Terre Haute, IN: Wish Publishing.

Edlin, G., & Golanty, E. (2007). *Health and wellness.* Boston: Jones and Bartlett.

Karinch, M. (2002). *Diets designed for athletes.* Canada: Human Kinetics.

Leeds, M. J. (1998). *Nutrition for healthy living.* Boston: WCB McGraw-Hill.

Litt, A. (2004). *Fuel for young athletes: Essential foods and fluids for future champions.* Champaign, IL: Human Kinetics.

Pearson, J., Goldklang, D., & Striegel-Moore, R. (2003). Prevention of eating disorders: Challenges and opportunities. *International Journal of Eating Disorders, 31,* 233-239.

Polivy, J., & Herman, C. (2002). Causes of eating disorders. *Annual Review of Psychology, 53,* 187-213.

Stice, E., & Shaw, H. (2004). Eating disorder prevention programs: A meta-analytic review. *Psychological Bulletin, 130,* 206–227.

Chapter 6

Aetna InteliHealth Inc. (2005). *Who needs supplements?* Retrieved March 12, 2006, from http://www.intelihealth.com/IH/ihtIH/WSIHW000/325/7098/34069.html?d=dmtContent.

The American Orthopaedic Society for Sports Medicine. (1993). *Anabolic steroids and growth hormone.* Retrieved March 13, 2006, from http://ajs.sagepub.com/cgi/ content/abstract/21/3/468.

Cool Nurse. (2000–2005). *What steroids can do to you: An article for parents and teens.* Retrieved March 13, 2006, from http://www.coolnurse.com/steroids.htm.

Duke University, Division of Student Affairs. (n.d.). *Energy bars.* Retrieved December 19, 2006, from, http:// healthydevil.studentaffairs.duke.edu/health_info/Energy%20Bars.html.

FDA/Center for Food Safety and Applied Nutrition. *Qualified health claims—Label claims.* Retrieved March 13, 2006, from http://www.cfsan.fda.gov/~dms/lab-qhc.html.

FindArticles. (2006). *Ergogenic Aids: Powders, pills and potions to enhance performance.* Retrieved March 13, 2006, from http://www.findarticles.com/p/articles/mi_m3225/is_5_63/ai_71267978-.

Johnson, C. (2006). *Some truth on energy bars: Students and a nutritionist weigh in on the positive and negative sides of these small, popular food items seen in many hands.* Retrieved December 19, 2006, from *The Daily Texan* Web site: http://www.dailytexanonline.com/home/index.cfm?event=displayArticlePrinterFriendly&uStory_id=1e8d0e5a-1b84-4c66-be98-a840ea52a27d.

The National Center for Drug Free Sport, Inc. (2006). *Drugs and sports.* Retrieved December 12, 2006, from http://www.drugfreesport.com.

The National Center for Drug Free Sport, Inc. (2006). *Human-growth hormone—The "secret boost"?: Lack of a test may make high the drug of choice.* Retrieved December 19, 2006, from http://www.drugfreesport.com/insight.asp?VolID=33&TopicID=7.

The National Collegiate Athletic Association. (2003). *NCAA drug-testing results.* Retrieved April 20, 2005, from http://www1.ncaa.org/membership/ed_outreach/health-safety/drug_testing/0203results.html.

The National Collegiate Athletic Association. (2005). *NCAA drug testing program website.* Retrieved December 11, 2006, from http://www1.ncaa.org/membership/ed_outreach/health-safety/drug_testing/index.html.

The National Institute on Drug Abuse (NIDA). (2005). *What are anabolic steroids?* Retrieved March 13, 2006, from http://www.nida.nih.gov/ResearchReports/Steroids/anabolic steroids2.html#what.

Searle, J. *Muscle medicine makes minds minuscule.* Retrieved March 13, 2006, from http://dsc.dixie.edu/barry/fall98/searlemuscle.htm

Smith, L. (Ed.). (2005). *The latest buzz training and conditioning.* Retrieved March 13, 2006, from http://www.momentummedia.com/articles/tc/tc1502/buzz.htm.

The University of Arizona, Department of Nutritional Sciences. (2002). *Ergogenic Aids.* Retrieved March 12, 2006, from http://ag.arizona.edu/NSC/new/sn/HPergogenic.htm.

Williams, M. H. (1996). Ergogenic aids: A means to citius, altius, fortius, and Olympic gold? *Research Quarterly for Exercise and Sport, 67,* 58–63.

Chapter 7

Harford, T. C., Wechsler, H., & Buthen, B. O. (2003). Alcohol-related aggression and drinking at off-campus parties and bars: A national study of current drinkers at college. *Journal of Studies on Alcohol, 64*(5), 704–711.

Kinney, J. (2006). *Loosening the grip: A handbook of alcohol information* (8th ed.). Boston: McGraw-Hill.

Kuo, M., Wechsler, H., Greenberg, P., & Lee, H. (2003). The marketing of alcohol to college students: The role of low prices and special promotions. *American Journal of Preventive Medicine, 25*(3), 204–211.

Levinthal, C. F. (2002). *Drugs, behavior, and modern society* (3rd ed.). Boston: Allyn & Bacon.

Powell, L. M., Williams, J., & Wechsler, H. (2004). Study habits and the level of alcohol use among college students. *Education Economics, 12*(2), 135–149.

Task Force of the National Advisory Council on Alcohol Abuse and Alcoholism. National Institutes of Health, U.S. Department of Health and Human Services. (2002). *High-risk drinking in college: What we know and what we need to learn: Final report of the panel on contexts and consequences.* Retrieved November 9, 2007, from "College drinking: Changing the culture," created by the National Institute on Alcohol Abuse and Alcoholism: http://www.collegedrinkingprevention.gov/media/FINALPanel1.pdf.

Wechsler, H., & Kuo, M. (2003). Watering down the drinks: The moderating effect of college demographics on alcohol use of high-risk groups. *American Journal of Public Health, 93*(11), 1929–1933.

Wechsler, H., Nelson, T. F., Lee, J. E., Seibring, M., Lewis, C., & Keeling, R. P. (2003). Perception and reality: A national evaluation of social norms marketing interventions to reduce college students' heavy alcohol use. *Journal of Studies on Alcohol, 64*(4), 484–494.

Wechsler, H., Seibring, M., Liu, I. C., & Ahl, M. (2004). Colleges respond to student binge drinking: Reducing student demand or limiting access. *Journal of American College Health, 52*(4), 159–168.

Weitzman, E. R. (2004). Social developmental overview of heavy episodic or binge drinking among U.S. college students. *Psychiatric Times, 2*(21).

Weitzman, E. R., & Nelson, T. F. (2004). College student binge drinking and the "prevention paradox": Implications for prevention and harm reduction. *Journal of Drug Education, 34*(3), 247–266.

Weitzman, E. R., Nelson, T. F., Lee, H., & Wechsler, H. (2004). Reducing drinking and related harms in college: Evaluation of the "A Matter of Degree" program. *American Journal of Preventive Medicine, 27*(3).

Wechsler, H., & Wuethrich, B. (2002). *Dying to drink: Confronting binge drinking on college campuses.* Emmaus, PA: Rodale.

U.S. Department of Health and Human Services, National Institutes of Health, National Institute on Alcohol Abuse and Alcoholism. (2003). *Alcohol: A women's health issue.* (Publication No. 03-4956). Retrieved November 9, 2007, from National Institutes of Health Web site: http://www.niaaa.nih.gov/NR/rdonlyres/57DD6ADD-6209-42BA-8831-754AD7580FBF/0/WomensBrochure.pdf.

Chapter 8

The Bacchus Network. (2002). *How to help a friend.* Retrieved January 5, 2007, from TobaccoFreeUniversity.Org Web site: http://www.tobaccofreeu.org/cessation/help_a_friend.asp#.

Canadian Cancer Society. (2007). *For smokers who want to quit—One step at a time.* Toronto, Ontario: Canadian Cancer Society. Retrieved October 29, 2007, from http://www.cancer.ca/vgn/images/portal/cit_86751114/8/18/1908600069OSAAT-Want_En_Booklet_2007.pdf.

Coombs, R. H., & Ziedonis, D. (Eds.). (1995). *Handbook on drug abuse prevention*. Needham Heights, MA: Allyn & Bacon.

Gangsta411.com. (2007). *Marijuana: A guide to quitting*. Retrieved January 5, 2007, from http://gangsta411.com/marijuana_a_guide_to_quitting.htm.

National Institute on Drug Abuse, National Institutes of Health, U.S. Department of Health and Human Services. (2006). *NIDA infofacts: Marijuana*. Retrieved November 9, 2007, from http://www.drugabuse.gov/PDF/InfoFacts/Marijuana06.pdf.

Smokefree.gov. (1994). *Online guide to quitting*. Retrieved January 5, 2007, from http://smokefree.gov/guide/basic_ steps.html.

University of South Florida, H. Lee Moffitt Cancer Center and Research Institute. (2000). *Forever free: A guide to remaining smoke free: An overview. Booklet 1 & 7*. Retrieved January 5, 2007, from http://www.moffitt.org/default.aspx.

Wadler, G. I., Hainline, B., & Ryan, A. J. (Eds.). (1989). *Drugs and the athlete*. Philadelphia, PA: F. A. Davis Company.

Chapter 9

AVERT. (2006). *Age of consent*. Retrieved April 19, 2006, from http://www.avert.org/age consent.htm.

Corey, G., & Corey, M. S. (2006). *I never knew I had a choice: Explorations in personal growth* (8th ed.). Belmont, CA: Thomson Brooks/Cole.

Curry, T. J. (1991). Fraternal bonding in the locker room: A profeminist analysis of talk about competition and women. *Sociology of Sports*, 8:119–135.

Curry, T. J. (1998). Beyond the locker room: Campus bars and college athletes. *Sociology of Sports*, 15:205–215.

Donatell, R. J. (2003). *Health the basics*. (5th ed.). San Francisco, CA: Benjamin Cummings.

Griffin, P. (1998). *Strong women, deep closets: Lesbians and homophobia in sport*. Champaign, IL: Human Kinetics.

Hahn, D., Payne, W., & Mauer, E. (2005). *Focus on health* (7th ed.). New York: McGraw-Hill.

Hendrick, S. S. (2004). *Understanding close relationships*. Boston: Pearson Education.

iVillage. (2006). *Sperm survival after ejaculation*. Retrieved April 19, 2006, from http://health.ivillage.com/infertility/0,,4pvn,00.html?iv_arrivalSA=1&iv_cobrandRef=0&iv_arrival_freq=1&pba=adid=15444627.

Messner, M. A., & Sabo, D. F. (1994). *Sex, violence and power in sports: Rethinking masculinity*. Freedom, CA: The Crossing Press.

Palo Alto Medical Foundation for Health Care. (2005). *Safer oral sex*. Retrieved April 19, 2006, from http://www.pamf.org/teen/sex/std/oral/.

Public Health Seattle & King Company. (2006). *Sexually transmitted diseases program*. Retrieved April 19, 2006, from http://www.metrokc.gov/health/apu/std/.

U.S. Department of Justice. (2005). *National crime victimization survey, violent crime trends, 1973–2003.* Retrieved April 19, 2006, from http://www.ojp.usdoj.gov/bjs/glance/tables/viortrdtab.htm.

Chapter 10

Bellringer, P., & Smeaton, M. (2003). *Types of gambling taken from need to know gambling.* Retrieved April 21, 2006, from GamCare Web site, http://www.gamcare.org.uk/site.builder/types.html.

The Common Sense Foundation. (1999). *Common sense says.* . . . Retrieved April 21, 2006, from http://common-sense.org/pdfs/css_v2_i04.pdf.

Foster, C., & Elliott, M. (2005). *Financial literacy for teens: The teen's guide to the real world of money.* Conyers, GA: Rising Books.

Gardner, J., Jewler, A. J., & Barefoot, B. (2007). *Your college experience: Strategies for success* (7th ed.). Boston: Thomson-Wadsorth.

Indiana University, Bloomington. (2006). *Sports gambling.* Retrieved April 24, 2006, from http://iuhoosiers.cstv.com/compliance/ind-compliance-gambling-sports-e.html.

Johnson, E. E., Hamer, R., Nora, R. M., Tan, B., Eisenstein, N., & Engelhart, C. (1997). The lie/bet questionnaire for screening pathological gamblers. *Psychological Reports,* 80(1):83–8.

National Collegiate Athletic Association. (2001). *Written testimony of William S. Saum, Director of Agent, Gambling and Amateurism Activities National Collegiate Athletic Association before the Judiciary Committee of the Nevada State Assembly.* Retrieved April 21, 2006, from http://www.ncaa.org/gambling/20010302_testimony.html.

National Collegiate Athletic Association (2004). *2003 NCAA national study on collegiate sports wagering and associated behaviors.* Retrieved November 8, 2006, from http://www.ncaa.org/library/research/sports_wagering/2003/2003_sports_wagering_study.pdf.

Chapter 11

Conley, D. (2005). *College knowledge.* San Francisco, CA: Jossey-Bass.

Ferrett, S. (2006). *Peak performance: Success in college and beyond.* Boston: McGraw-Hill.

Langan, J. (2003). *Ten skills you really need to succeed in college.* Boston: McGraw-Hill.

Nist, S., & Holschuh, J. (2006). *College success strategies.* New York: Penguin Academics.

University of Texas at El Paso. (2007). *Borders: Crossing into your future.* Plymouth, MI: Hayden-McNeil.

Worthington, J. F., & Farrar, R. (1998). *The ultimate college survival guide: Proven tips and techniques for success* (4th ed.). Lawrenceville, NJ: Thomson-Peterson.

Index

- Lewis Henry Morgan

- 1871 ... consanguinity ...

- ... Kinship

- US – Monogamy   one man one women   ...

- Polygamy – multiple
  - 1. Polygyny $O + \triangle = O$
  - 0. Polyandry $\triangle = O = \triangle$

- Group Marriage

  Ways of acquiring ...

  ... Bride Price (Progeny Price)

  Like buying ...